Signals and Communication Technology

This series is devoted to fundamentals and applications of modern methods of signal processing and cutting-edge communication technologies. The main topics are information and signal theory, acoustical signal processing, image processing and multimedia systems, mobile and wireless communications, and computer and communication networks. Volumes in the series address researchers in academia and industrial R&D departments. The series is application-oriented. The level of presentation of each individual volume, however, depends on the subject and can range from practical to scientific.

Indexing: All books in "Signals and Communication Technology" are indexed by Scopus and zbMATH

For general information about this book series, comments or suggestions, please contact Mary James at mary.james@springer.com or Ramesh Nath Premnath at ramesh.premnath@springer.com.

Suparna Biswas

Machine Learning and Deep Learning in Human Activity Recognition and Fall Detection

Algorithms, Frameworks, and Applications for Sustainable Healthcare

Springer

Suparna Biswas
Department of Computer Science
and Engineering
Maulana Abul Kalam Azad University
of Technology
Haringhata, West Bengal, India

ISSN 1860-4862 ISSN 1860-4870 (electronic)
Signals and Communication Technology
ISBN 978-3-032-09240-3 ISBN 978-3-032-09241-0 (eBook)
https://doi.org/10.1007/978-3-032-09241-0

This Springer imprint is published by the registered company Springer Nature Switzerland AG
The registered company address is: Gewerbestrasse 11, 6330 Cham, Switzerland

I am dedicating this book to my daughters
Rini and Bini

—Dr. Suparna Biswas

Preface

The topic to be illustrated and highlighted in this book is human activity recognition (HAR) and fall detection (FD) of human being remotely with the application of "smart" technologies as defined in Industry 5.0 such as wearable and smartphone sensors, Internet of things, cloud, machine learning, and deep learning for privacy-aware activity recognition of the people under monitoring. The activities in concern could be sit, stand, walk, run, stairs up, stairs down, jumping, jogging, laying, etc., as a human being undergoes during daily cores. The elderly people are living mostly alone without manual monitoring for a longer period of time due to socioeconomic scenario, to afford a manual monitoring support may always not possible, and also it hampers the privacy issue as well. Hence, by exploiting the available infrastructures like smartphone, WiFi, or Internet connectivity in urban and in developed rural areas, privacy aware, low cost, seamless activity, and fall monitoring could be done for identifying any abnormal posture or severe fall event in real time for necessary and timely support. The abnormal activities or sudden fall events identification will generate an alert message and will be sent to the registered mobile numbers of nearest relatives, caregivers, healthcare centers, ambulances, etc., for immediate support. Also every time a fall event gets detected, its immediate pre-fall posture or activity is also recorded to find a pattern of fall, and it would help to diagnose any specific disease the person is suffering from or is prone to suffer. If an elderly person is mostly falling down from pre-fall posture as stand or walk that indicates he might have gait problems or may be suffering from arthritis or may have sleep apnea or disorder that makes nerves, muscles of leg weak, etc., so, this book will highlight the application of HAR and fall detection in the disease prediction, disease detection, etc., and the appropriate recommendation of health expert's advice could be sought on time. To make the solutions smart and sustainable, advanced technologies such as machine learning, deep learning, wearable and smartphone sensors, Internet of things, and cloud are being utilized to avail efficient and cost-effective solutions. Sensor fusion, data fusion, and information fusion-based techniques are used to analyze, process multimodal data collected through heterogeneous sensors. The data, processing, activity, and fall detection-related methodologies, prototypes, etc., are well illustrated to quench the thirst of the readers and to ignite the interested minds to explore further through the whole book in this challenging research domain.

Salient Features of the Book

- **What interesting aspects for the readers?** This book is a combination of fundamental concepts, case studies, prototype demonstration while utilizing sensor, IoT, cloud, machine learning, deep learning, artificial intelligence, sensor fusion, etc., in different applications along with detailed addressing to the issues related to performance evaluation, privacy issues, etc.
- **Target Audience:**
    i. **Undergraduate and Postgraduate Students:** Exposure on HAR and fall detection frameworks with challenges and opportunities is given to the students studying computer science and engineering and allied fields.
    ii. **Researchers:** To be enriched with the innovative research motivations that could be addressed in different problems discussed.
    iii. **Faculty members:** This book can be used by the faculty members as a reference book on different aspects such as design, development, analysis, problem identification, solving on sensor-based HAR, FD applying ML and DL-related applications.

Case Studies

Extensive case studies have been illustrated highlighting implementation perspectives, prototype development, and prototypes that are being used in practice, etc., to have an idea of the achievability of the advanced HAR and FD systems.

Structure

This book provides a holistic journey toward interested readers. Chapter 1 is introduction to human activity recognition, fall monitoring and detection, health monitoring, elderly care, smart and sustainable healthcare frameworks, healthy living, etc., with detailed illustration. Chapter 2 describes fundamental concepts, introduction and overview of enabling smart technologies—sensors, Internet of things, machine learning, deep learning, and cloud technologies. Chapter 3 is detailing on machine learning models in human activity recognition using smartphone sensor, fundamental concepts of machine learning, smartphone as sensor hub, accelerometer sensor, gyroscope sensor, machine learning models in HAR, application of accelerometer and gyroscope data in HAR, and datasets analysis. Chapter 4 depicts deep learning in human activity recognition using smartphone sensors deep learning models, automatic feature extraction, and datasets for deep learning-based HAR. Chapter 5 is focused on application of machine learning in fall detection system, machine learning-based fall detection models, frameworks, fall detection with pre-fall posture recording for disease prediction that are well illustrated. In Chap. 6, sensor fusion-based HAR for disease monitoring and prediction, sensor fusion concept, wearable and smartphone sensor data fusion for HAR, FD, health monitoring and care, etc., are mainly elaborated. Chapter 7 brings the interesting part to readers by exploring through few design, development, deployment strategies, prototypes, case studies, scenarios-based studies, etc. Chapter 8 concludes the whole book by summarizing all the contributions, highlighting unique features of this book to the readers and highlight of future scope.

Haringhata, India Suparna Biswas

Acknowledgements I would like to express my sincere thanks and gratitude to all those who contributed to the writing and development of this book. I would also like to thank my research scholars and research team, my department and my university for their valuable insights and support. Also, I am thankful to my beloved daughters, family members for their unconditional support to successfully complete this endeavor. To be very specific in acknowledgement, Dr. Suparna Biswas wants to acknowledge her university, department, and her research team in her Internet of Things Lab comprising of UG, PG students and Ph.D. scholars. On machine learning, deep learning in HAR and fall detection, contributions of Dr. Pratik Bhattacharjee and Ms. Pragya Sharma are being thankfully acknowledged. Dr. Dipanwita Thakur awarded with Ph.D. degree on HAR has progressed significantly with HAR-related research using ML and DL. This book aims to be a valuable resource for anyone interested in learning about and utilizing sensors, IoT, cloud, ML, DL in HAR, and FD. We hope that it will inspire readers to explore the vast possibilities of this exciting technology and contribute to its further development.

Competing Interests The author has no competing interests to declare that are relevant to the content of this manuscript.

About This Book

This book provides a complete knowledge resource to the interested readers and budding researchers to get acquainted with the domain of human activity recognition and fall detection of people specifically elderly people for seamless monitoring and support. This HAR and FD have immense application in disease monitoring, prediction and identification as well in real time facilitating early diagnosis of symptom-based disease identification, prediction, detection, etc., exploiting existing infrastructure support ecosystem comprising of smartphone, WiFi, 3G/4G Internet connectivity, low cost wearable sensors, etc., for sustainable health monitoring and care. Smart technologies such as machine learning, deep learning, and Internet of things are applied for sensor data analysis and knowledge extraction toward accurate identification of activities and fall events with pre-fall postures in real time. Human activity recognition along with fall detection has immense application in sustainable health monitoring and care targeted for elderly care. Also this system could be used as a confidence building tool to the diseased elderly suffering from age-related ailments such as Parkinson's, Alzheimer's, gait problems, heart diseases, and sleep apnea. The smart and seamless health monitoring and care ecosystem would only be complete with such smart monitoring systems along with traditional healthcare system for sustainable solution.

Contents

1 Introduction 1
1.1 Introduction 1
1.2 Human Activity Recognition (HAR) 2
1.3 Fall Detection and Monitoring (FDM) 2
1.4 Health Monitoring (HM) 4
1.5 Elderly Care or Geriatric Care 5
1.6 Smart and Sustainable Healthcare Frameworks 7
1.7 Why and How "Sustainable"?? 10
1.8 How to Detect Fall Event? 11
1.9 Sustainable HAR Frameworks 13
1.10 Privacy-Preserving HAR 15
1.11 The Properties of Context-Awareness and Being Adaptive of HAR Systems 17
1.12 Open-Source HAR Platforms 18
1.13 Conclusion 22
References 22

2 Fundamental Concepts of HAR 25
2.1 Introduction and Overview of Enabling Smart Technologies 25
2.1.1 What are Enabling Technologies of a Smart System or Application? 25
2.1.2 What are the Enabling Technologies Required in Smart and Intelligent Human Activity Recognition? Why these are called "Enabling Technologies"? 25
2.1.3 Sensors Used in HAR 28
2.1.4 Vision-Based Sensors 32
2.1.5 Hybrid Sensor Systems 33
2.1.6 Data Preprocessing 33
2.1.7 Feature Selection and Dimensionality Reduction 36

2.1.8 Internet of Things as Enabling Technology in HAR and Health Care ... 37
2.1.9 Machine Learning in HAR ... 38
2.1.10 Unsupervised Machine Learning ... 41
2.1.11 Deep Learning-Based Methods ... 42
2.1.12 Key Advantages of Using Edge Computing in HAR ... 44
2.1.13 Cloud Computing in HAR ... 45
2.2 Conclusion ... 46
References ... 47

3 Machine Learning in Human Activity Recognition ... 49
3.1 Introduction ... 49
3.2 State-of-the-Art Literatures: A Comprehensive Study ... 50
3.2.1 Sensors Used ... 50
3.2.2 Data Preprocessing ... 55
3.2.3 Classification ... 57
3.2.4 Design of an Activity Monitoring System ... 59
3.3 Performance Metrics ... 60
3.3.1 Challenges and Future Directions in HAR ... 60
3.3.2 Data Collection and Annotation Challenges ... 61
3.3.3 Sensor Heterogeneity and Fusion ... 62
3.4 Real-Time Processing and Computational Constraints ... 62
3.4.1 Privacy and Ethical Considerations ... 63
3.4.2 Emerging Trends and Open Research Questions ... 64
3.5 Conclusion ... 65
References ... 66

4 Deep Learning in HAR ... 69
4.1 Introduction ... 69
4.2 Types of Deep Learning Models Used in HAR ... 71
4.2.1 Convolutional Neural Networks (CNNs) ... 71
4.2.2 Recurrent Neural Networks (RNNs) ... 72
4.2.3 Long Short-Term Memory (LSTM) Networks ... 74
4.2.4 Gated Recurrent Units (GRUs) ... 75
4.2.5 Deep Belief Networks (DBNs) ... 76
4.2.6 Autoencoders ... 77
4.3 Convolutional Neural Networks (CNNs) Used for HAR-Related Disease Detection ... 78
4.3.1 Parkinson's Disease Detection Using DaTscan Images ... 78
4.4 Datasets for Human Activity Recognition Applied with Deep Learning Techniques ... 79
4.4.1 UCI HAR Dataset and Deep Learning Models ... 79
4.4.2 MobiAct Dataset and Deep Learning ... 79

4.5 Automatic Feature Extraction in Human Activity Recognition Using Deep Learning 80
4.5.1 Convolutional Neural Networks (CNNs) 80
4.5.2 Recurrent Neural Networks (RNNs) and LSTM 81
4.5.3 Autoencoders 81
4.5.4 Hybrid Models (e.g., CNN-LSTM) 81
4.6 Conclusion 82
References 83

5 Machine Learning in Fall Detection Systems 87
5.1 Introduction 87
5.1.1 Sensor Technologies and Data Acquisition 87
5.1.2 Preprocessing and Feature Extraction 88
5.2 Supervised Machine Learning for Activity Recognition 89
5.2.1 Classification Algorithms 89
5.2.2 Model Training and Validation 90
5.3 Fall Detection Architectures 90
5.3.1 Threshold-Based Triggers 90
5.3.2 Hybrid Threshold–ML Systems 90
5.3.3 End-to-End System Integration 91
5.4 Fall Risk Analysis and Prediction 91
5.4.1 Timed Up-and-Go (TUG) Test Metrics 91
5.4.2 Grip Force and Gait Symmetry 91
5.4.3 Multimodal Risk Models 92
5.5 System Evaluation and Benchmarking 92
5.5.1 Datasets and Protocols 92
5.5.2 Performance Metrics 92
5.5.3 Comparative Results 92
5.6 Challenges and Future Directions 95
5.7 Conclusion 95
References 96

6 Sensor Fusion-Based HAR for Disease Monitoring and Prediction 97
6.1 Introduction 97
6.2 Challenges in HAR 98
6.3 Information Fusion 98
6.4 Sensors in Sensor Fusion for Activity Recognition 100
6.4.1 Smartphone Sensors 100
6.4.2 Feature Extraction 100
6.4.3 Classification 100
6.4.4 Advantages of Accelerometers in HAR 101
6.4.5 Why Accelerometer and Gyroscope give better Performance when Combined? 101

6.5 Data Fusion ... 102
6.5.1 Example of Data Fusion Using IMU Sensors in HAR ... 102
6.5.2 Sensor Fusion ... 103
6.6 Sensors Used in Various Fusion Methods for HAR, Fall Detection, and Healthcare Applications ... 106
6.6.1 Sensors in HAR and Fall Detection ... 106
6.7 Multimodality in Sensor Fusion ... 108
6.7.1 Case Study 1: FamilyLog ... 108
6.7.2 Case Study 2: WMMS ... 109
6.8 Conclusion ... 109
References ... 110

7 Design and Prototypes of HAR and FD Systems ... 113
7.1 Introduction ... 113
7.1.1 Using Sensor, IoT, and Cloud—Most Popularly Explored in HAR and FD for Health Care ... 114
7.1.2 Using Radar Technology for Health Care—Less Explored Pathway ... 115
7.2 Datasets Used in HAR ... 119
7.2.1 Key Issues in HAR Datasets ... 119
7.3 Datasets Used in Human Activity Recognition (HAR): Description and Comparative Analysis ... 121
7.3.1 Fall Datasets ... 121
7.4 Case Studies and Scenario Based on HAR Systems ... 125
7.4.1 Channel Status Information (CSI)-Based HAR ... 125
7.4.2 Smartphone-Based HAR ... 125
7.4.3 RADAR-Based Fall Detection (FD) System ... 126
7.4.4 Prototype Components ... 126
7.4.5 Sensor Fusion-Based HAR ... 127
7.5 Scenario-Based Study ... 127
7.6 Reference Sensor Attached to the Environment-Based Human Activity and Movement Recognition ... 128
7.6.1 Wearable Sensor-Based HAR ... 128
7.6.2 Fall Detection Scenarios ... 131
7.7 Conclusion ... 134
References ... 134

8 Conclusion ... 137

Index ... 145

About the Author

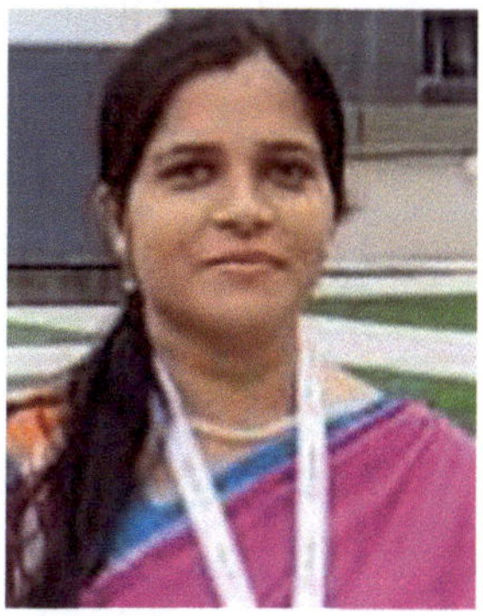

Dr. Suparna Biswas is working as an associate professor in the Department of Computer Science and Engineering in Maulana Abul Kalam Azad University of Technology, West Bengal. She has received M.E. and Ph.D. from Jadavpur University, West Bengal. She has been an ERASMUS MUNDUS postdoctoral research fellow in cLINK project in Northumbria University, Newcastle, UK. She has successfully completed two funded research projects in the capacity of PI and Co-PI in the area of smart health care using WBAN, IoT. She has co-authored a research book on adhoc and sensor network. She has successfully guided 6 Ph.D. research scholars in the broad domain of IoT-based health care and network security, 80 UG, and 40 PG final year projects. She has been the lead editor in publishing edited book, has been lead organizing chair, session chair, session organizer in the international conferences, etc. She is a technical committee member of many international conferences of repute and has served as a reviewer in reputed journals, conferences, etc. She has delivered a number of invited lectures in seminars, workshops, webinars, FDPs and invited tutorial lectures in international conferences. She has published more than 100 research papers published in reputed journals with good indexing and high impact factors including Q1 journals in association with national and international collaborations, in international conferences, and as book chapters of repute. She has been granted with two international patents for innovation in development of a Smart Health Monitoring Assistance prototype for Parkinson's diseased people, and as recognition the work has been published in leading National Newspaper as well. She has 20 years of teaching experience and is teaching subjects like Internet of things, machine learning, Internet of things security, network security, etc. Her areas of research interests are Internet of things, machine learning, smart healthcare, precision agriculture, network security, etc. She had executed administrative responsibilities as the head of the department during 2020–2022, various administrative committee members at University level, department level etc. She has been a university MOOCs coordinator and is SPOC of NPTEL-SWAYAM of MAKAUT, West Bengal, since 2017. She has organized seminar, training, workshop, AICTE-funded ATAL FDPs, and MeitY funded FDPs as a coordinator etc. She is a senior member of IEEE.

Chapter 1
Introduction

1.1 Introduction

Gesture is defined as body parts movement to signify or express any speech more clearly. And human activity is a combination of gestures, actions, and interactions, etc., over a period of time. Human activities could be static and dynamic, simple and complex, e.g., SITTING, STANDING, LAYING are static and simple activities, WALKING is simple but dynamic, RUNNING, JOGGING, JUMPING, STAIRS UP, STAIRS DOWN, etc., are dynamic and complex activities. In dynamic activities, body parts have temporal movement, such as JOGGING. In some class of activities, whole body along with body parts' temporal movement continues, such as RUNNING, WALKING, and STAIRS UP. These activities mentioned here so far are performed for daily cores, almost by all the people at any time during day and night, irrespective of gender, age, economic condition, health condition (except a person is old, diseased, unable to move, etc.), etc.

There are some activities which are mainly household activities such as COOKING, IRONING, WASHING CLOTHES, WASHING DISHES, MOPPING, DUSTING, and CLEANING. These are complex, dynamic activities mostly performed at day time and mostly by women, specifically in developing countries and rural areas. These activities are very complex, dynamic activities and can be difficult to label with high accuracy. To enhance accuracy in identification of complex human activities, role of intelligent algorithms such as machine learning and deep learning is very much important.

Now, the big questions roaming around ignited minds are manifold:

1. How to recognize human activities/postures remotely maintaining privacy?
2. What are application domains/areas to apply this knowledge?
3. How to ensure real-time recognition of activities for utilizing in time-critical applications?

S. Biswas, *Machine Learning and Deep Learning in Human Activity Recognition and Fall Detection*, Signals and Communication Technology,
https://doi.org/10.1007/978-3-032-09241-0_1

4. What are the crucial issues and challenges in implementing such systems in mass usage for people specifically for senior citizens?

All questions will be well explained and answered in details in subsequent readings. For now in brief first question will be explained.

1.2 Human Activity Recognition (HAR)

Prior to get detail knowledge on any domain or topic, we must be aware of its evolution history or background. When people first thought of this human activity recognition (HAR) as a research problem? What had been the driving force behind it? How this would have been implementable in real-life problem solving toward enhanced quality living? Is HAR still in research and experimental status or in use by general people?

While we will read through this chapter, we will come to the answers gradually.

The very first research paper on human activity recognition (HAR) has been published in 90s [1, 2]. Till date a large number of works have been done and published. The driving force behind this continuous research in the domain of HAR is the urge to improve accuracy in recognition of dynamic, complex activities in real environment with given conditions and here lies the challenges.

Few of these challenges are as follows:

(a) The attributes—The features to be selected and measured.
(b) The data collection module—An efficient, low cost, user friendly, seamless data collection systems or module development is still a challenge.
(c) Feature engineering—Feature extraction from complex, dynamic, unlabeled activities, feature selection, or optimization for dimension reduction is a continuously hammered area of research.
(d) Data engineering—In realistic, dynamic environment, collection of data is a real challenge.
(e) The flexibility to support new users without the need of re-training the system, and the implementation in mobile devices meeting energy and processing requirements [3].

1.3 Fall Detection and Monitoring (FDM)

Another point of concern while we talk about human activity recognition is about fall event which is sudden and can prove to be fatal if not recognized and supported immediately for recovery. People specifically elderly suffering from age-related ailments such as Parkinson's, Alzheimer's, gait issues, diabetes, hypertension, and sleep apnea are prone to frequent and sudden fall both at indoor or at outdoor. If this fall event is left unrecognized and unattended, then that could be life threatening as well. The elderly live mostly alone without manual monitoring, and they want to live normal life supported with independent mobility due to daily cores at indoor as well as outdoor like morning walk, going to market or medicine shop or hospital, etc. But if they suffer from sudden, frequent fall and that is not recognized and supported for recovery in time, and then they may lose their confidence for leading normal life with necessary movement. So fall monitoring and detection for timely support to the people in concern specifically elderly people is significantly required to ensure quality living in confidence. For both HAR and FDM, the very common question or query would be how these can be achieved with ensured accuracy? Just to introduce with the concept, these are monitored and recognized with the help of advanced enabling technologies such as sensors, Internet of things, machine learning, deep learning, artificial intelligence, and cloud. Primarily the sensors collect the human motion or movement-related raw data, and Internet of things transmits these raw data to the cloud server, machine learning, deep learning, artificial intelligence, neural network-based intelligent, complex models for processing big, sensory data to recognize specific activity or fall event. Now the question comes, how human activity recognition (HAR) and fall detection (FD) are connected or related to each other when it comes to the problem to address on ensuring quality life of people specifically elderly providing support of a smart, intelligent assistance along with traditional systems such as health monitoring and care.

The Relation Between HAR and FD

Laying and sitting are human activities which may indicate both normal or abnormal health and physical condition of a subject based on specific context.

When Normal?

Posture: Laying, sitting.

Immediate Pre-posture: For laying–sitting, for sitting–standing.

Context

Location: Indoor or outdoor, at indoor at bedroom or drawing room. At outdoor, sitting at park, medicine shop, restaurant, etc., normal but laying at these locations is considered as abnormal activity.

Duration: At day time, sitting duration is more than laying, but at night time, laying duration is more than sitting.

When Abnormal?

Context

Location: Indoor or outdoor, at indoor if the location is bathroom or kitchen or balcony or dining table, at outdoor on road or roadside, in a field, etc.

Duration: At day time, sitting is less, laying time more and at night, just opposite.

Now again, these scenario-based apprehensions of normal or abnormal activities may change in different context and will be described in detail in subsequent readings.

Immediate Pre-posture: For laying and sitting may also be considered as abnormal based on the context of immediate pre-posture, this abnormal condition will be treated as fall based on this context. For example, for laying and sitting, if pre-posture activity was walking, running, jumping, jogging, stairs up or stairs down, etc., then this event would be a fall event.

The fall detection is a research wing that is done using motion sensor data analysis, and also detecting immediate pre-posture activity for a particular posture could lead to detection of fall event.

1.4 Health Monitoring (HM)

Now, with the continuation of previous topics of HAR and FDM, the combined ultimate purpose is health monitoring. Here we need to understand how health monitoring is associated or can be achieved through HAR and FDM. First we need to just precisely know what is the purpose of health monitoring? Health monitoring helps to sense human health vital parameters and analyze those data remotely to evaluate the health condition of the human being. Now, consider a scenario: A person at indoor or at outdoor suddenly falls down. The FDM module will detect fall event and generate an alert for necessary support and recovery. The HAR module will recognize current posture/activity and immediate pre-posture/activity. If pre-posture and current posture combination is abnormal as discussed earlier, then this will also report a fall event and will generate an alert. Now, with biomedical sensors wearable or implanted in human body forming wireless body area network or medical body sensor network (MBSN), the biological parameters in general being sensed are body temperature, blood pressure, heart rate, pulse rate, oxygen saturation, blood sugar level, etc., and if any one or more of these parameters are found to be in abnormal or critical range as per medical definition, then also an alert will be generated for appropriate medical support.

Now, if we see these three modules of HAR, FDM, and HM, individually they may fail to identify a health scenario of a person as abnormal or critical one and generate alert to exert support in time.

Scenario: A person only falls down due to stumble or bad road condition or collision with other person or any obstacle due to unmindful walking, etc., and can recover on his own, then it seems to be quite a normal scenario, not a scenario to generate alert, and here lies the grave health concern.

How FDM looks at it? FDM detects it as a fall event and generates alert, if recovery detection module (RM) is not associated with FDM.

How HAR looks at it? HAR recognizes it as a fall event by combining posture and pre-posture and generates alert.

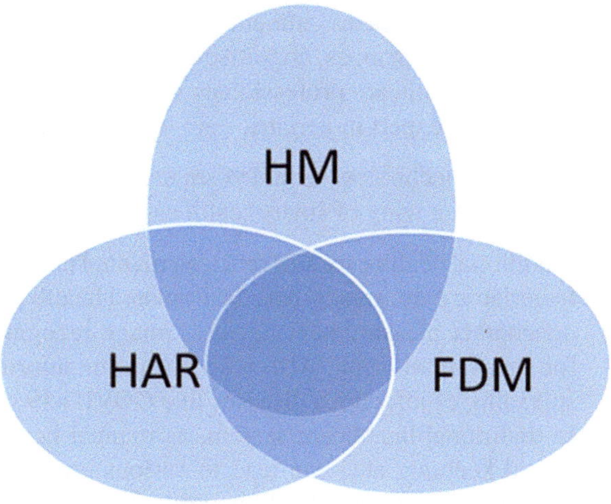

Fig. 1.1 Health care completes with health monitoring, human activity recognition, and fall detection module

How HM looks at it? If all vital health parameters are within normal range as per medical definition within this fall and recover event duration, then it is a normal health condition scenario. But if any of the health parameters are in abnormal or critical range, then appropriate medication should begin.

Another flaw in HM could be, if the general health parameters are unable to detect any health abnormality which could be possible reason of fault, then this health abnormality remains unrecognized. For example, if the person is having sleep apnea or sleep disorder [4], gait issue and appropriate sensors are not in MBSN for monitoring such diseases, then these can trigger fall events with immediate self-recovery, not causing severe fall, then this abnormality will remain unrecognized by HM module and by all three modules, as already explained. Such events if are ignored for long period of time can cause serious health issues development causing gait at severe level, sleep disorder-related diseases such as Alzheimer's and Parkinson's. So, total health care (HC) will comprise all three modules to complete the circle as shown in Fig. 1.1.

1.5 Elderly Care or Geriatric Care

"Healthcare sector that cares about changing needs of elderly people, specifically provides mental, physical, social, and cognitive support to develop an ecosystem comprising trained healthcare professionals, advanced technologies, etc., to automate the process of health monitoring, wellness monitoring, medical treatment for age-related ailments, etc., to ensure a healthy, independent, confident, mobile, and quality living of the elderly is called geriatric care".

So, geriatrics or gerontology is a domain of research in health care that deals with:

1. Physical, mental, sociological, and cognitive support to the elderly

2. Age-related diseases, ailments, and physical and mental disability support
3. Sociological changes, cognitive imbalance-related support
4. To train healthcare professionals with appropriate knowledge, tools, techniques to become expert in geriatric care to extend support to the elderly.

Now, why technology-enabled smart, automated geriatric care has come up as a special separate wing of smart health care? The reasons behind are manifold:

- Traditional health care still relies on manual health vital parameters measurement. In geriatric care, sensor-based automated health parameter collection and distant, noncontact measurement devices, image recognition techniques, etc., are used for smart monitoring. Also with distant monitoring and measurement facilities, spreading of infectious diseases like COVID-19 could also be restricted.
- In traditional healthcare system, as manual health data collection, paper-based record keeping, etc., can lead to various errors. Manual error in health parameter measurement and health record collection may be missed, regularity of data collection may not be maintained accurately, health data, pathological test reports, medical advices, diagnosis, etc., are still paper-based and may not be kept properly sequence wise to the hospital or the patient. Thus, the continuous treatment, referring back to background medical history with health data and records, etc., may not always be in place. For prolonged treatment of age-related ailments such as Alzheimer's, Parkinson's, COPD, heart-related diseases, stroke patients, and diabetes, referring back to history of patient condition and treatment, diagnosis, etc., are very much important.
- For age-related diseases that demand prolonged regular routine treatment cycle of pathological tests, reporting and visiting a doctor, medication and again pathological tests at an interval as advised and again visiting the doctor physically. This cycle goes on and on demanding an accompanying person, time, travel expense, effort in appointment booking, if the patient or the accompanying person is in rural areas then long hours of travel, etc. These could be avoided in many cases and situations if it is a routine checkup, follow-up, and only analyzing body vitals on regular basis, doctor can advise proper medication and treatment from remote end. Number of physical visits in this way may be reduced or minimized.
- Not only for ongoing treatment, but for rehabilitation purpose also, the appropriate record keeping of health data and medical history are very much significant. In geriatric care, all health data, pathological reports, doctor's prescription, diagnosis reports, etc., are stored as electronic health record (EHR) so that as and when required, could be accessed, referred, analyzed to find the health issue patterns, past recovery rate, response at rehabilitation process, etc.

Figure 1.2 shows the geriatric care as a subset of smart health care as geriatric care is all about elderly health care to ensure seniors' quality living.

It is a multidisciplinary or interdisciplinary research wing that involves doctors, nurses, pathologists, biologists, technologists, data analyst, psychologist, sociologist, etc., to exert an ecosystem for the elderly combining the knowledge of all these fields.

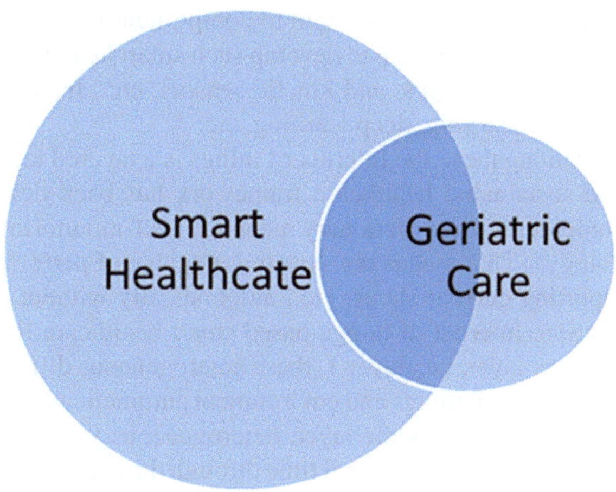

Fig. 1.2 Geriatric care—a special type (subset) of smart health care

To collect health data with sensors, devices, to transmit data seamlessly to cloud server for storing, analysis of data for knowledge generation, to access data as and when required, etc., combination of various technologies are applied.

(i) Data collection: Sensors, health devices
(ii) Data aggregation: Sink or coordinator or gateway devices
(iii) Data transmission: Heterogeneous communication links, short range, long range
(iv) Data storage and analysis: Cloud server
(v) Data analysis models: Machine learning, deep learning
(vi) Output data access: Smartphone applications (Android-based apps)
(vii) Alert generation, emergency message access: Smartphone.

Data collection through large number of biomedical sensors, data transmission through heterogeneous links, and data processing at cloud server combines to the advanced 3-tier revolutionary technology known as Internet of things (IoT).

1.6 Smart and Sustainable Healthcare Frameworks

Health care is a sector that is required by all human being in this world, irrespective of age, gender, economic, social status, location, or habitat. Now, the traditional healthcare system is inadequate in terms of health establishment infrastructure, healthcare professionals, manual monitoring, record keeping problems, etc. Also, to visit the doctor physically at regular intervals for routine checkup in case of prolonged treatment of age-related diseases such as diabetes, heart disease, hypertension, Parkinson's, and Alzheimer's, may always not be possible for the patient, and this will hamper the treatment and recovery process. So, to overcome all such obstacles, a smart healthcare and recommendation system will work in parallel with the traditional healthcare system to compliment it for better service. And the advanced technologies that help to develop such smart healthcare system are wearable sensors, biomedical sensors, and kinetic sensors, etc., Internet of things, cloud computing, machine learning, deep learning, etc.

Among these the Internet of things is a layered technology based on which smart and sustainable healthcare framework has been developed. "Smart" is a word in computer science dictionary meaning "self-monitoring, analysis, and reporting technology". That means the system is capable of performing monitoring, analysis, and reporting current status, etc., automatically without or with minimal human intervention. Internet of things-based smart healthcare framework is shown in Fig. 1.3. In lower layer, i.e., layer 1, these heterogeneous different kinds of sensors sense data from physical things and environment automatically at frequent and regular intervals. In layer 2, i.e., middle layer, heterogeneous various kinds of communication links transmit sensor data in real time through the edge devices like gateway nodes, routers, etc., that do the data aggregation, elementary preprocessing like denoising, discarding redundant or junk data, etc. In upper layer, i.e., layer 3, the data is transferred to cloud server for storage, processing applying complex, intelligent models enabled with machine learning, deep learning, artificial intelligence, etc. After processing the extracted and generated knowledge, data, information is accessed by authorized entity ensuring data privacy and security. After generated knowledge or feedback, if actuation process is required like any control in physical environment needs to be done, that is also done automatically. In all the processing, no or minimal manual intervention is required.

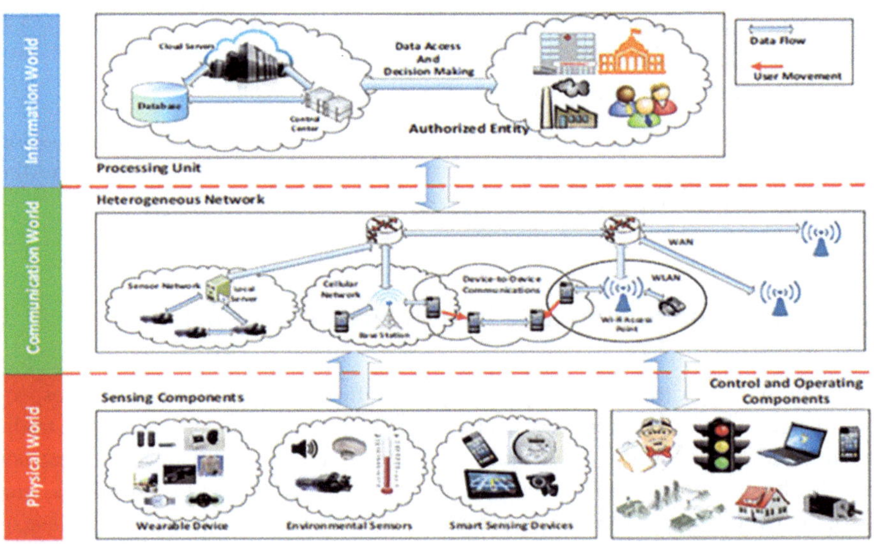

Fig. 1.3 Layered Internet of things framework for data sensing, transmitting, storage, and processing

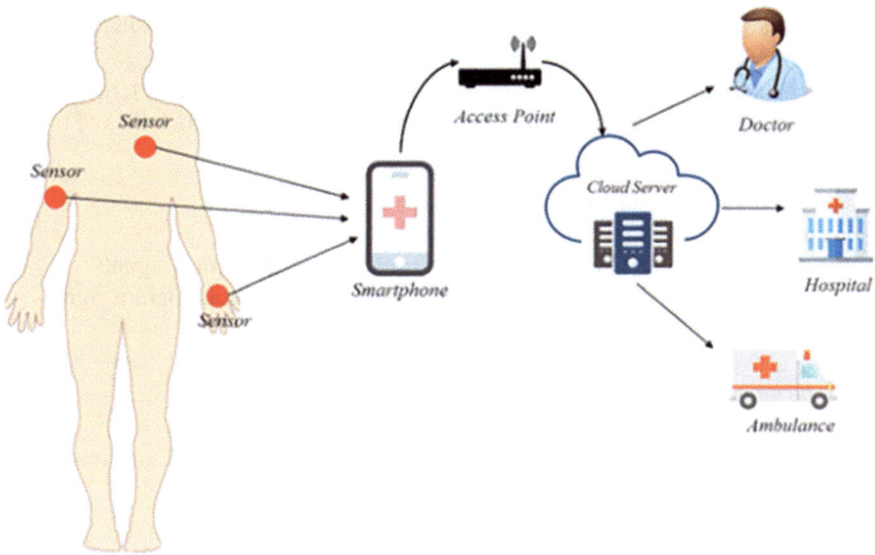

Fig. 1.4 MBSN sensor, IoT, cloud-based 3-tier architecture of smart health care

Here, in Fig. 1.3, the smart healthcare framework can sense data, transmit, analyze, generate patterns, etc., for health monitoring, fall detection, disease detection, prediction, etc.

Now in Fig. 1.4, specifically in the scenario of smart and sustainable health monitoring and care system is depicted. The biomedical sensors are spread over the human body, may be wearable or implanted, gathering body vital parameters and sending to the cloud over the Internet, 3G/4G connectivity. Biomedical sensors are connected with heterogeneous communication links such as Bluetooth BLE, WiFi, and Zigbee for medical body sensor network.

After health data is being processed at cloud server, doctors, nurses, hospital, or any other concerned stakeholder can access for necessary immediate action.

Now the things need to be clearly explained are as follows:

How this sensor, IoT, cloud, machine learning, deep learning-enabled health monitoring, and care system as described so far is (i) Smart, (ii) Sustainable!!

Why and How "Smart"??

Generally traditional health monitoring means monitoring of health condition of a person through monitoring vital health parameters. That is generally done by being measured through some devices at doctor's place being in certain physical proximity of the doctor/nurse, measurements could be of blood pressure, blood sugar, body temperature, pulse rate, oxygen saturation level (SpO_2), etc. And if some pathological tests required, then sample collection at pathological lab, or USG, ECG, etc., all need to visit pathological lab physically, and then report collection and again visiting the doctor for advice completes 1 treatment cycle. In all steps, human intervention is required.

Now in technology-enabled healthcare system as depicted in Fig. 1.4, these health vitals collected could be automated through biomedical sensors as follows [1, 2]:

- Temperature sensor to measure body temperature
- Blood pressure sensor to measure blood pressure
- Heart rate sensor that measures heart rate
- Electrocardiogram (ECG) sensor to measure electrocardiogram signals
- Electroencephalogram (EEG) sensor to record electroencephalogram signals
- Respiration rate sensor that measures respiration rate
- SpO_2 sensor that measures SpO_2 levels
- Blood sugar level sensor that measures blood sugar level
- Triaxial accelerometer sensor to detect human motion, activity
- Bend and respiratory flow sensors: Sensors that measure bend and respiratory flow
- GPS sensor: A sensor that can identify subject's location.

The health vitals based on health conditions will be recorded and sent over IoT to the cloud to be accessed by the doctor at remote end and accordingly advice, medicines or based on health condition patient may be advice for physical checkup, or any specialized pathological tests and diagnosis or even hospitalization. So, initial regular health monitoring will go on automatically at regular intervals without any manual intervention—thus this system is "SMART".

1.7 Why and How "Sustainable"??

Any system or service is said to be sustainable when it is long lasting, user friendly, accurate, economic, and having societal benefit at large. The technology-enabled smart health monitoring and care system of which human activity recognition and fall detection is a part is having all the characteristics of being sustainable. The reasons behind are as follows:

- The smart system is long lasting as it is coming up as a parallel system of the traditional health monitoring and care system.
- This is user friendly as the patient's vitals parameters are being collected and sent to the doctor without physical movement of the patient to the doctor's place, and doctor's advice is also reached to the patient at his own place—through wearable sensors, usable, and less expensive over all, hence usable.
- The sensors sense vital parameters automatically, without manual intervention, and hence there is no manual error, at regular interval.
- Wearable IoT-enabled biomedical sensors would be utilized for health data collection for prolonged time, and sending data is done utilizing existing WiFi or Internet connectivity at patient's location. Also the expense to travel to the doctor's place,

to go to diagnostic center or pathological laboratory, etc., will be saved. Overall the solution is economic to afford.

- As the elderly people get less mobile with increasing age at body and mind, due to age-related diseases, proneness to fall or being alone most of the time, they lose confidence. Hence, if a solution for primary health support enabled with advanced technologies could be assured, then quality of living would be increased.

1.8 How to Detect Fall Event?

Now the question that must be around is how human activity recognition can be done and what to do with this knowledge?

Basically almost all of us are having smartphone which is carried by us almost all the time attached to our body parts, e.g., carried in hand, in pant or shirt pocket, in waist position in belt, in ladies bag, etc. And the smartphone is a sensor hub having more than 50 sensors. Different types of sensors in a smartphone are as follows:

- Motion sensors such as accelerometer, gyroscope
- Gravity sensor
- Curve vector sensor
- Location sensor
- Environmental sensor
- Position sensor
- Magnetometer sensor
- Physiological sensor.

Accelerometer and gyroscope together form IMU unit in which accelerometer measures liner movement and its acceleration over 3-axis: along *X*, *Y*, and *Z* axes. The angular velocity is measured by gyroscope sensor, i.e., **rotation around *X*, *Y*, and Zaxes**. Smartphones, smartwatches, and wearable devices are nowadays commonly embedded with these IMU sensors.

A fall event can be described in a more elaborate manner by sketching it as a combination of three phases:

1. When the person is doing some static or dynamic activity like sitting, standing, lying, walking, running, etc., and becomes unstable due to some reason like getting stumble at some obstacle in walkway, or getting misbalanced from current activity or may due to abnormal physiological parameter like blood pressure or blood sugar levels, the person gets physically imbalanced—physical imbalance or instability.
2. The mid-phase after phase 1 and before complete fall is when the person feels sudden body acceleration or sudden rotation. Before complete fall down on a surface, the mid-phase where the fall is happening is called mid-phase or phase 2 of fall event, and here **sudden acceleration and/or rotation of the body happen**.

3. This is the last and final phase in which fall event has completely occurred, the subject or the person becomes immobile or inactive due to impact of sudden fall—post-fall phase.

These three different fall phases actually register different pattern of accelerometer and gyroscope data to distinctively identify these different three phases of fall event.

Fall detection systems work on two different working principles:

1. Threshold-based method
2. Machine learning-based method.

Threshold-Based Methods

This method works on the principle that the accelerometer reading if exceeds a certain value or level then within a very short time period then this event gets registered as a fall event. This method is immensely popular due to its simplicity, easy to implement, low cost, and affordable solution in terms only utilization of a smartphone in appropriate way. For real-time processing, the threshold-based method is preferred over other methods because due to its simple and easy processing steps, it can ensure real-time processing of the fall event, and it is very much required because fall is a time-critical and sometimes life-critical event. During free fall, a sharp spike is detected, and the acceleration value if would be more than 2 g or less than 0.5 g, then a sharp spike gets detected as a free fall. Another measurement that helps in detecting fall event is through capturing body rotation. With the help of gyroscope sensor, by monitoring the rapid changes in body rotation during a fall, fall can be distinguished from normal daily activities, which often involve slower, more controlled movements. Gyroscopes measure the rate of change of angular orientation (rotational acceleration). A fall involves a sudden, uncontrolled rotation of the body, which the gyroscope can detect as a spike in angular velocity. Normal activities like walking, sitting, or even jumping involve specific patterns of rotational movement. A fall, however, is characterized by a distinct, rapid, and often erratic rotation that differs significantly from these patterns. While gyroscopes excel at detecting rotational changes, accelerometers are better at sensing linear acceleration and impact forces. Combining data from both sensors provides a more comprehensive and accurate picture of the event, allowing for better differentiation between falls and other activities. As fall is a sudden, uncontrolled event, its after impact or post-impact of fall is almost very low or no movement for a few seconds. If this sudden body rotation is recorded during fitness regime or exercise session or yoga session, then the movement or body rotation will be fast but in a controlled manner, and post-impact will be immediate movement or with few seconds. In essence, the gyroscope's ability to precisely measure body rotation, combined with the accelerometer's ability to measure linear acceleration, enables the creation of robust fall detection systems that can significantly improve safety for individuals at risk of falling.

Threshold-based fall detection module (pseudocode):

If acceleration sensor value is less than 0.5 g (i.e., detection is free fall)
AND acceleration more than 2 g within 1 s (to evaluate the impact)
AND gyroscope sensor reading reflects high angular velocity
AND if very low or no motion for post 2–5 s (post fall impact)
Then → "Fall has occurred"

Machine Learning-Based Method

As sensory data is large and different other sensors are also coming into the picture leading to sensor fusion method or concept, to build up knowledge based using different unique features, machine learning-based methods gained immense popularity and efficiency. From raw accelerometer sensor data or accelerometer and gyroscope combined data, different features are extracted for model training purposed with training dataset. The input features are mean, variance, max, min, energy, jerk, etc. Once the training with sufficient labeled data is done and model hypothesis gets developed, then the testing and validation continue. Different machine learning models such as SVM, random forest, CNN, and LSTM are being efficiently and popularly being used in state-of-the literatures.

The dataset may consist of only accelerometer data or combination of accelerometer or gyroscope data and the application could be for only HAR or HAR and FD for making the system suitable to the elderly care. The works on HAR and fall monitoring are ever evolving and ever improvising from the point of view of reducing falls positives or true negatives so that reliability of the system could be enhanced. From that point of view, sensor fusion is being applied primarily combining accelerometer or gyroscope data. For example, accelerometer records movement or motion and its impact, whereas the rotational movement is detected through gyroscope sensor to avoid or reduce instances of false positives. Practical scenario if we consider like if a person is doing some exercises and he is doing push-ups or sit-ups. In sit-up, as person's move is very fast sitting, this may be wrongly detected as fall. Advanced systems use sensor fusion techniques like Kalman filters or deep learning models to integrate data from both.

1.9 Sustainable HAR Frameworks

Sustainable Development or Solution

Sustainable development aims for solutions to be used in long term without disturbing or causing harm to the future generation's need or causing imbalance or hazards to the surrounding environment or ecosystem. Sustainable frameworks ensure standard practices, tools, techniques, methodologies to be used that ensure reliability, scalability, robustness, usability, affordability of the solution along with balancing economic growth, social equity, environmental protection, etc.

Here we are concerned about sustainable frameworks for **human activity recognition (HAR)** that not only aims to ensure best performance of the system in recognizing specific human activity but maintains some of the important properties or characteristics of the system that make it sustainable as follows:

1. Energy-efficient
2. Privacy-preserving
3. Reliable
4. Scalable
5. Affordable
6. Usable
7. Values and ethics.

What best practices are followed to ensure energy efficiency in HAR systems? Some of these are as follows:

Utilization of TinyML

When Machine learning algorithms are deployed on resource-constrained devices having limited memory, bandwidth, processing power, energy source, the solutions may be infeasible to execute in long term etc. Generally in human activity recognition, data collecting devices are smartphones, smart watches, fitness trackers embedded with IMU sensors, i.e., accelerometers and gyroscope. Now if sensory data as collected by the motion sensors of the smart devices can be analyzed or processed at the device itself for activity detection or recognition, then its benefit is many-fold ensuring sustainability:

1. Sensory data need not to be sent to the cloud, thus saving energy consumption
2. Ensures real-time activity identification
3. Reduces latency or end-to-end delay
4. Maintains privacy.

Utilization of TinyML by deploying machine learning models on microcontrollers allows for local computations on wearable devices locally without sending them to cloud, thus saves resources, and makes the framework sustainable.

- **Key Role Played by Edge Computing**

If the sensory data is processed at the edge devices, i.e., on microcontrollers of the smart device itself, then the need to send data to the cloud gets minimized, and in effect, energy consumption gets reduced. Also latency, i.e., from the time instance of raw sensor data collection to the time instant of activity recognition is the latency or the delay considered here. This delay gets much reduced if data gets processed at edge end.

- **Increased Accuracy with Personalized Models**

Training HAR models on user-specific data can lead to more accurate and efficient activity recognition, reducing the need for computationally expensive generalized models.

HAR Solution with Energy Efficiency

Goal: To minimize power consumption because this is specifically important for battery operated smartphone or any other smart, wearable HAR devices. Now what are the different mechanisms or methods that could be followed to ensure low power consumption? Sensing is the main task that provides the raw data upon which the techniques to be applied. And sensing is done by huge number of sensors at a very frequent rate or interval. And this sensing, transmission, receiving of data, processing, etc., demand huge power consumption at sensor level or at processing unit may be at edge end or at cloud end. Most of the sensors, edge devices are battery operated. Hence, if energy consumption could be controlled and limited at this level, then the system could be more sustainable.

Techniques Used

Techniques applied are as follows: Utilization of low power sensors such as:

- Use of accelerometers, gyroscopes over camera sensors, i.e., utilizing low power hungry sensors.
- Sensors will be doze mode, and receiver radio antenna will be in sleep mode unless and until there is any motion or movement—then only sensors will be active, and data collection will take place, i.e., to ensure data collection triggered by event or there is a significant change in motion.
- Raw sensory data once collected needs to be processed in real time and for that options is to process them closure to the point of origin to ensure low latency or reduce communication cost or to transmit data to the cloud end through long-range communication link such as 3G/4G. So, for priority or emergency data that needs to be analyzed for knowledge or pattern generation and to raise alert or take necessary action in minimum delay, edge computing is always a preference over cloud computing.
- And final processing stage is to train the model with preprocessed data, and if lightweight ML models can be chosen, e.g., TinyML, pruning, quantization, etc., then overall energy requirements of the end-to-end system could surely be ensured.

1.10 Privacy-Preserving HAR

Motion or movement or activity data is a personalized data that demands privacy, i.e., to be used by or revealed to only legitimate ones. Some required additional measures may be taken to ensure privacy. If the computation or processing or the HAR framework is ensuring this, then this is a privacy-preserving framework. Obvious goal of such frameworks is to protect user data and to ensure ethical use of personal activity information. There are several popular and efficient approaches that enhance privacy of HAR systems. Some of these are as follows:

- Privacy or security threats to the raw sensory could take place at different stages of HAR system—could be at sensor layer or at short-range communication link using Bluetooth, WiFi, Zigbee connecting between sensor and edge device or at long-range communication link, 3G/4G or at edge devices or at cloud server—any point could be attack point. If the raw data processing could be done in a privacy-aware fashion like using federated learning, then ML models could be trained across multiple devices without transferring raw data.
- Always it may not be possible to avoid transmitting raw sensory data including identity, personal credentials of individuals over open wireless channel through 3G/4G Internet connectivity, sometime to confuse with the attackers, noise could be added to data to prevent stealing of identification credentials of the individuals—this technique is called differential privacy.
- If privacy-sensitive data could be processed at local end, i.e., at user's device without transmitting the data to the remote end, then also privacy of data could be ensured—the power of smart devices could be exploited for this purpose.

Scalable and Transferable Models

One of the primary requirements of sustainability is to make the system scalable and transferable to cope up with future need. This is associated with sustainability because these make HAR system independent of environment, type or number of users, and the underlying context based on which the system will work. The efficient and popular techniques that are widely applied are as follows:

- **Using transfer learning model**: This can ensure scalability by developing the pretrained models by training on large datasets and then continuing with fine-tuning for specific applications.
- **By ensuring domain adaptation**: This means if there is change or updating in sensor setup being used or in the users of the system, then the models can adjust and cope up with the changes ensuring performance level.
- **Multimodal fusion**: Combine data from multiple sources (e.g., audio, motion, and GPS) for robustness.

Environmental and Social Sustainability

Sustainability is not complete without ensuring environmental and social sustainability. Now what are the different aspects of environmental sustainability or how the HAR system could be made environ friendly? In HAR, a large of smart wearable devices are generally used by large number of users. Now, the devices often may give erroneous functionalities or no functionalities demanding repairing or discarding of the sensors or devices like smart watches with accelerometer, gyroscope sensors, fit bit sensors, and smart wearables such as in the form band or belt or spectacle or ring or shirt. Now if these could be manufactured with eco-friendly or recyclable materials, then discarding of these devices will not cause any environmental harm. Another aspect is for social sustainability, we must ensure or look into the matter by taking necessary measures to ensure digital equity. Now what is digital equity and how it could be assured? Providing low cost solution and to achieve that we need to utilize and chose technologies that would ensure low cost solutions so that the HAR systems could be affordable at under privileged regions as well. And smartphone-based HAR systems are best example of this low cost solution for sustainability, due to Digital India project almost all people of our nation is having smartphone and unlimited data in their possession, and if this could be exploited to develop the system, then obviously the system will be sustainable in long term. Smartphone-based solutions or applications are always preferred by users irrespective of their age group, abilities, sociocultural status, etc. So basically tow properties, i.e., eco-friendly devices and digital equity could be the significant factors to develop environmental and social sustainability in HAR systems.

1.11 The Properties of Context-Awareness and Being Adaptive of HAR Systems

The goal of these properties is to enhance performance, reduce power consumption, reduce computational complexity, etc., to ensure improvement in efficiency and reduction in data collection that are unnecessary. And to implement and achieve these, the system could be made customization to be adaptive to the controlling factors such as sampling rate, user feedback, and smart scheduling of HAR in sync with device idle time. Now how the sampling rate is associated? The sampling rate could be adaptive instead of fixed based on type of activity, e.g., static versus dynamic activities have different nature and frequency of change in acceleration. In activities like sit, stand, sleep versus in activities like walk, run, etc., the sampling rate could be made adaptive, not making flat or fixed. Also user feedback could be involved in accurate predictions by the devices by giving options to them to validate the prediction by either directly correcting them or influencing them in any method. HAR devices are battery operated, and they go to sleep of or snooze or doze mode while not active to save battery power. Now the HAR application that is implemented in the device itself could be made to work in such as manner so that it works in sync with the device idle time to save power. So the features in summary that could make the HAR system to be context-aware and adaptive are as follows:

- **Adaptive sampling rates**
- **User feedback integration**
- **Smart scheduling.**

Use of Open Data and Standardization

In HAR-based works reported so far, many of the systems have been developed promoting open-source HAR frameworks and shared public datasets to encourage reproducibility and collaborative improvements. Developing common benchmarks and evaluation standards help to compare HAR systems fairly.

1.12 Open-Source HAR Platforms

There are several open-source HAR platforms that support real-time, privacy-preserving HAR data analytics, and some of these are given below:

- **OpenHAR**: Open-source HAR platform supporting real-time, privacy-aware analytics.
- **TensorFlow Lite + Edge TPU**: Enables sustainable deep learning for HAR on edge devices.
- **AWARE Framework**: Mobile context instrumentation for energy-aware HAR.
- **Sustainable AI Frameworks**: Focused on green AI practices (e.g., Carbontracker, and CodeCarbon for ML energy profiling).
- **BodyFlow**: A comprehensive library that seamlessly integrates human pose estimation and multiple-person estimation and tracking, along with activity recognition modules.
- **Apple Watch Fall Detection**
- **AAL (Ambient Assisted Living) Projects in the EU**
- **MIT AgeLab Smart Home Sensors**
- **Eldercare-Focused Datasets**: e.g., *MobiAct*, *SUS-ADL*, and *Opportunity*.

Figure 1.5 shows an overview of sustainable HAR frameworks, addressing both technological and socioenvironmental aspects.

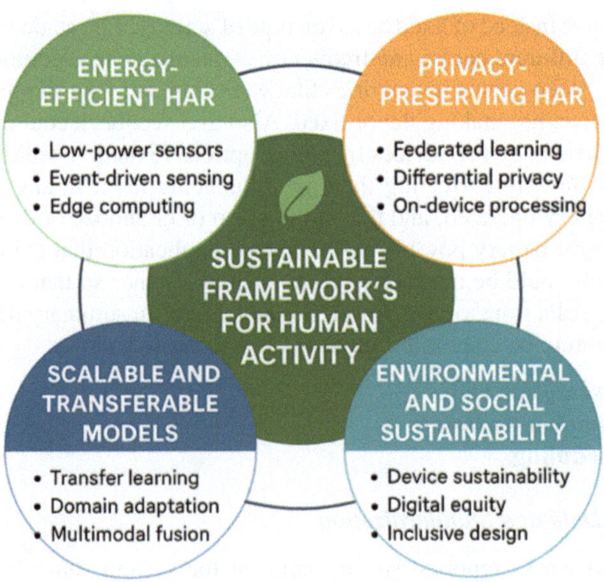

Fig. 1.5 Representative framework of sustainable human activity recognition

The diagram effectively communicates the multidimensional nature of sustainability in HAR systems, combining technical, ethical, and ecological components. The diagram in Fig. 1.5 represents 4 quadrants:

Top Left Quadrant

Top left quadrant represents energy efficient HAR in terms of

- **Sensors with low power consumption property**
- **Sensing only when some trigger event occurs**
- **Sensory data processing at edge devices.**

This section emphasizes reducing energy consumption during data collection and processing.

Top Right Quadrant

The top right quadrant of the diagram in Fig. 1.5 is highlighting the **privacy-preserving requirement in HAR. Several popular techniques that are used to ensure privacy are as follows**:

- **Federated learning**
- **Differential privacy**
- **On-device processing.**

This quadrant focuses on protection of personalized HAR data from being exposed to illegitimate entities and preventing privacy breached through implementing distributed learning and efficient local data handling.

Scalability of such frameworks in one of the very important characteristics of making the HAR system sustainable for long because in near future either for fitness tracking, or for household chores monitoring or for elderly people's monitoring, fall detection, etc., more and more number of users will get added to the system.

The Bottom Left Corner

This quadrant represents scalable and transferable models of the framework. The techniques that are efficiently applied to ensure scalability in such frameworks are as follows:

- **Transfer learning**
- **Domain adaptation**
- **Multimodal fusion.**

This quadrant focuses or elaborates on different properties such as flexibility, model reusability, and adaptability across diverse environments or on the user contexts.

Last Bottom Right Corner

This quadrant is the last bottom-right quadrant that reflects on sustainability in terms of Environmental and Social aspects. This quadrant deals with following salient features:

- **Device sustainability**
- **Digital equity**
- **Inclusive design**.

Human Activity Recognition (HAR) in Elderly Care: A Detailed Description

Human activity recognition (HAR) is a rapidly growing area of research and application in health care, particularly for supporting elderly care. It involves the use of sensors and machine learning algorithms to automatically detect, monitor, and analyze human actions such as walking, sitting, sleeping, or falling.

Why HAR Is Important in Elderly Care

As per report of WHO, elderly population is alarmingly increasing, and this is global scenario. Due to socioeconomic changes, most of them are living either alone, unattended most of the day time or under the manual observation or monitoring. Here, the sensory human activity recognition and fall detection system plays a pivotal role. Elderly people may be suffering from chronic diseases or may not, but due to aging effect, bone and muscle decay or weakness, or foot imbalance problem, they are prone to fall [5]. Here automated and continuous fall monitoring and timely support help them to perform their daily activities necessary for living may be both at indoor and at outdoor [6, 7]. As the global elderly population increases, many seniors live alone or require continuous supervision due to:

- **Age-related mobility issues**
- **Chronic diseases** (e.g., Parkinson's and dementia)
- **Risk of falls and accidents**
- **Cognitive impairments**.

HAR systems offer a **nonintrusive and automated solution** to monitor their well-being and safety in real time.

How HAR Works in Elderly Care

HAR works amazingly and efficiently well in elderly care as it has been discussed in the previous sections, in geriatric care part as well. Here the step-by-step working of HAR-based elderly care is shown below (Fig. 1.6):

- **First Step: Sensor Deployment**

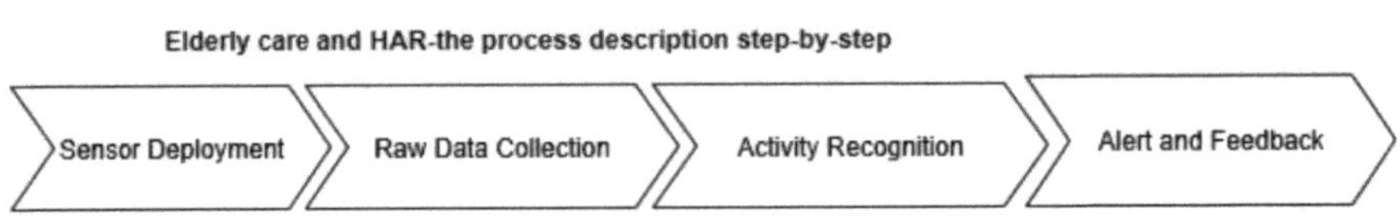

Fig. 1.6 Elderly care and HAR workflow

Sensors could be heterogeneous acquiring heterogeneous data and leading tot sensor fusion or data fusion to enhance accuracy. Different types of sensors mainly used are wearable sensors: Smartwatches, pendants, or belts equipped with accelerometers, gyroscopes, and heart rate monitors. Ambient sensors: Motion detectors, cameras, pressure mats, or microphones placed in the home environment. Smartphones/ Tablets: Leverage built-in sensors and apps to monitor activity.

- **Second Step: Data Collection**

Sensor data is time-series data and may be collected in continuous or periodical fashion. This processing step includes pattern of movement of the user, different activities or postures, specific location of the user, and vital physiological signals (heart rate, pulse rate, temperature, blood pressure, breathing rate, etc.).

- **Third Step: Activity Recognition**

To analyze sensor data for pattern identification and knowledge extraction, intelligent and efficient machine learning (ML) or deep learning (DL)-based models are applied [8]. In this process step, detection or classification of activities in different classes is performed like sitting, standing, lying, walking, jogging, jumping, stairs up or down, sleeping, cooking, or any sudden fall event or stumble, etc., is done with high accuracy and efficiency.

- **Fourth Step: To generate Alerts and Feedback**

This is the most crucial stage of whole process, and this step ensures that proper action is taken by the respective concerned authority based on the activity class recognized in the previous step. If a fall or anomaly is detected, [9] real-time alerts can be sent to caregivers or emergency services. Dashboards or mobile apps allow family members or doctors to monitor activity trends.

HAR benefits elderly people to gain real-time monitoring and care which are as shown in Table 1.1.

Table 1.1 Description of factors by which elderly care gets benefited using HAR

S. No.	Benefit	Description
1	Fall detection	Immediate alerts for accidents can reduce time to treatment
2	Health monitoring	Tracks alerts for accidents can reduce time to treatment
3	Independence	Encourages again in place with reduced need for constant supervision
4	Caregiver support	Reduces burden on healthcare provider and family members

1.13 Conclusion

This chapter basically describes basic fundamental concepts of human activity recognition and fall detection systems using heterogeneous sensors wearable or embedded in smart devices such as smartphones, smart watches, and Fit-bits [10–12]. HAR and FD systems have various applications aimed for enhancing quality living and societal benefit specifically for the elderly for monitoring and extending support in real time may be at indoor or at outdoor. [13–16] This introduction chapter actually introduces interested readers and researchers with the basic components of HAR systems, frameworks, architectures, different methodologies being used, application domains, sustainability issues for long-term applications, how HAR and FD is useful tool for elderly care improving quality of their life, etc. This chapter gives a holistic view to the readers to begin with and to inculcate their curiosity, to quench their thirst to know more on the data collection, models to be applied, actual system development and deployment in real-world scenario, case studies, scenario-based description, etc., are there in subsequent chapters.

References

1. El-Adawi, E., Essa, E., Handosa, M., et al. (2024). Wireless body area sensor networks based human activity recognition using deep learning. *Science and Reports, 14*, 2702. https://doi.org/10.1038/s41598-024-53069-1
2. Darwish, A., & Hassanien, A. E. (2011). Wearable and implantable wireless sensor network solutions for healthcare monitoring. *Sensors (Basel), 11*(6), 5561–5595. https://doi.org/10.3390/s110605561. Epub 2011 May 26. Erratum in: *Sensors (Basel), 12*(9), 12375–12376 (2012). PMID: 22163914; PMCID: PMC3231450.
3. Schlmilch, O. X., Witzschel, B., Cantor, M., Kahl, E., Mehmke, R., & Runge, C. (1999). Detection of posture and motion by accelerometry: A validation study in ambulatory monitoring. *Computers in Human Behavior, 15*(5), 571–583.
4. Stevens, D., Jackson, B., Carberry, J., McLoughlin, J., Barr, C., Mukherjee, S., Oh, A., McEvoy, R. D., Crotty, M., & Vakulin, A. (2020). The impact of obstructive sleep apnea on balance, gait, and falls risk: A narrative review of the literature. *Journals of Gerontology. Series A, Biological Sciences and Medical Sciences, 75*(12), 2450–2460. https://doi.org/10.1093/gerona/glaa014. PMID: 32039438.
5. Gaud, N., Rathore, M., & Suman, U. (2024). MHCNLS-HAR: Multi-headed CNN-LSTM based human activity recognition leveraging a novel wearable edge device for elderly health care. *IEEE Sensors Journal.*
6. Schrader, L., Vargas Toro, A., Konietzny, S., Rüping, S., Schäpers, B., Steinböck, M., et al. (2020). Advanced sensing and human activity recognition in early intervention and rehabilitation of elderly people. *Journal of Population Ageing, 13*(2), 139–165.
7. Bibbò, L., Carotenuto, R., & Della Corte, F. (2022). An overview of indoor localization system for human activity recognition (HAR) in healthcare. *Sensors, 22*(21), 8119.
8. Human fall detection and activity monitoring: a comparative analysis of vision-based methods for classification and detection techniques. ACM Publication.
9. A comprehensive review of elderly fall detection using wireless communication and artificial intelligence techniques.

10. Foerster, F., Smeja, M., & Fahrenberg, J. (1999). Detection of posture and motion by accelerometry: A validation study in ambulatory monitoring. *Computers in Human Behavior, 15*(5), 571–583.
11. Kim, E., Helal, S., & Cook, D. (2010). Human activity recognition and pattern discovery. *IEEE Pervasive Computing, 9*(1), 48–53.
12. Khan, A. M., et al. (2014). Human activity recognition on smartphones using a multiclass hardware-friendly support vector machine. *Sensors*.
13. Lane, N. D., et al. (2015). DeepX: A software accelerator for low-power deep learning inference on mobile devices. In *IPSN*.
14. Xu, C., et al. (2021). Sustainable edge AI for human activity recognition. *IEEE Internet of Things Journal*.
15. Gao, Y., et al. (2020). Privacy-aware human activity recognition from low-resolution videos. In *ECCV*.
16. del-Hoyo-Alonso, R., Hernández-Ruiz, A. C., Marañes-Nueno, C., López-Bosque, I., Aznar-Gimeno, R., Salvo-Ibañez, P., et al. (2024). BodyFlow: An open-source library for multimodal human activity recognition. *Sensors, 24*(20), 6729.

Chapter 2
Fundamental Concepts of HAR

2.1 Introduction and Overview of Enabling Smart Technologies

2.1.1 What are Enabling Technologies of a Smart System or Application?

Enabling technologies help in execution and conduction of a system to be smarter and efficient in terms of minimum manual intervention, automated data monitoring at regular intervals, efficient data handling, extracting meaningful information about the system, and intelligent solution in real time with ensured privacy and security.

2.1.2 What are the Enabling Technologies Required in Smart and Intelligent Human Activity Recognition? Why these are called "Enabling Technologies"?

Enabling technologies are the technologies that aid the smooth functioning of the system by helping in computation of fundamental tasks in efficient and intelligent manner.

In human activity recognition system, the following are the key tasks:

- Automated human motion data collection—Enabling Technology: Kinematic motion sensors such as accelerometer and gyroscope, wearable or smartphone sensors or in smart watch.
- Data Transmission—Enabling Technology: Communication links such as WiFi, Bluetooth, and Zigbee.

S. Biswas, *Machine Learning and Deep Learning in Human Activity Recognition and Fall Detection*, Signals and Communication Technology,
https://doi.org/10.1007/978-3-032-09241-0_2

- Data aggregation and preprocessing—Edge devices such as sink device, coordinator device, and gateway device.
- Data transmission for storage and processing—Sensory data is transmitted to cloud server through long-range communication technology such as LTE.
- Processing of sensory data or physical data—Intelligent, complex models using ML, DL, AI, etc., are applied for data processing at cloud server for knowledge extraction.
- In case of any emergency health condition or event such as Fall, stroke etc., the event will be detected and alert message or advice of healthcare expert in case of health emergency would be sent to the registered mobile number of the person in concern.

To ensure all these primary real-time communications, smartphone-based applications development helps as an enabling technology by applying appropriate protocols, frameworks, tools, technologies, programming languages, etc.

1. To enable devices to function reliably and efficiently, embedded system helps, and if the smart devices (mainly sensors, smartphones, edge devices, cloud infrastructure, etc.) function properly with accuracy, precision, timeliness, etc., then the smart applications must function efficiently and appropriately in real-time manner.

Table 2.1 illustrates different enabling technologies as discussed so far starting from sensors to cloud to embedded and communication technologies and specific tasks performed by each of these enabling technologies applicable to HAR, FD, etc., and corresponding specific technology components.

2.1.2.1 Sensors

Sensors are ears and eyes of any modern day smart application. Sensors are devices tiny in size, lightweight, and can collect or detect changes in the physical environment. The change can be measured as it would be converted to measurable signal, mostly electrical signal.

Definition: A **sensor** is a device that can gather data or change in data in physical phenomenon such as temperature and light intensity and convert into signal in the form of voltage and current that can be measured.

Sensors have varying properties or features that make them of different types, and some of the important properties are as follows:

- **Accuracy**: How close is the measured value with the actual one
- **Range**: The limit of the physical parameter a sensor can correctly measure
- **Response Time**: The time by which the sensor can react to the change in the environment
- **Resolution**: The ability of a sensor to detect smallest change in the physical environment

Table 2.1 Enabling technologies in HAR and fall detection

S. No.	Enabling technologies	Tasks in smart HAR, and fall detection	Specific technology components
1	Sensors	Kinematic motion data sensing and collection from the subjects	Transceiver unit, power supply, and sensing and actuation unit
2	Communication links	Short-range and long-range communications for sensor data transmission to the cloud server	WiFi, Bluetooth, Zigbee, etc.
3	Edge devices	These devices aggregate, preprocess, and transmit data from sensor to the edge device and edge device to the cloud server	Smartphone, gateway, switch, router, laptop computer, tablet computer etc.
4	Cloud server	Big sensory data storage, processing and results storage, and results accession by the authorized entities	Private, public cloud servers
5	Intelligent models	Big sensory data analysis by the intelligent models for knowledge generation, meaningful information extraction, etc.	Machine learning, deep learning, artificial intelligence, and neural networks
6	Smartphone-based APPLICATION Development (APP)	To send alert messages, send necessary advice to the stakeholders in time etc.	Android APP Development
7	Embedded technologies	To enable devices to function reliably and efficiently	Sensors, smartphones, edge devices, and cloud infrastructure

- **Sensitivity**: It is the ratio of the change in output signal change to input signal change.

Based on types of parameters to be measured, applications to be developed in which the sensors to be used, power requirement, material used in the sensor, etc., sensors could be of many types.

This chapter presents an overview of sensors and their classifications as thermal, magnetic optical, mechanical and chemical, and also their applications on different real-life applications.

Sensors in Mobile Phones Used in Health Care

The health monitoring sensor, also known as bio-sensors, is a self-contained analytical device which includes a biologically active substance (triggered by sound, light, motion, etc.) in close contact with a suitable transduction component to detect (reversibly and selectively) the density or movement of substances in a sample. The common mobile phone sensors that can be used for health monitoring are listed below.

Microphone Sensor

The feel of the patient may be assessed using a microphone sensor, e.g., patients having the myotonic syndrome. Myotonia is a type of disorder categorized by sluggish relaxation of muscles after contraction that can result in a trouble in movement. The patients need to inform their heath data by calling the data collection center within 8 weeks of consultation.

An automated voice response scheme identifies symptoms into four categories: muscle stiffness, weakness, pain, and tiredness [2].

Camera Sensor

Telemedicine and remote physician consultations involve utilizing the mobile phone's camera sensor to gather valuable data from images and videos of patients through a dedicated application. This approach is particularly applicable in the realm of teledermatology, where doctors leverage patient skin images for diagnostic purposes. The capabilities of the mobile device's camera can be expanded by integrating additional specialized components with the phone. Motion sensors such as accelerometer sensor and GPS sensor are also embedded in smart home and can be used to design various activity/motion/movement monitoring application s of human being. Accelerometers can be utilized to find movement pattern and to evaluate movement ability of a patient who may be suffering from chronic diseases [3]. Additional special sensors such as SpO_2 and temperature along with accelerometer, gyroscope, and GPS sensor have made it possible to design applications related to patient monitoring with location information exploiting the smartphone only.

2.1.3 Sensors Used in HAR

Primary task in HAR is data collection which is primarily wearable sensor based in most of the literatures: Sensors used are described below.

2.1.3.1 Data Acquisition Using Wearable Sensors

Data collection is the very first step of any human activity recognition system since the quality and suitability of the harvested data influence the accuracy and stability of activity recognition directly. HAR systems use a wide range of sensors with varying abilities to capture different aspects of human motion and interaction with the world. These sensors can be broadly classified according to their deployment and sensing modality.

Wearable sensors are arguably the most ubiquitous and natural option for HAR, as they are attached directly to or worn on the subject, offering intimate and continuous body kinematic and physiological state measurements. Their close proximity to the activity source facilitates the collection of fine-grained, high-fidelity data, rendering them essential for numerous HAR applications. HAR applications are utilized in health monitoring, health care, geriatric care solutions as well [4].

2.1.3.2 Inertial Measurement Units (IMUs)

Inertial measurement units (IMUs) are sensor combinations that are normally composed of accelerometers, gyroscopes, and occasionally magnetometers. They are common in contemporary smartphones, smartwatches, and specialized wearable devices, serving as the core component of a majority of HAR systems because they have the capacity to record detailed motion dynamics.

i. ***Accelerometers***: An accelerometer detects nongravitational acceleration, or proper acceleration, of the device. For HAR, accelerometers usually acquire linear acceleration on three orthogonal axes (X, Y, and Z). This information is essential to identify changes in speed, direction, and orientation. From patterns in acceleration, one can even recognize walking, running, jumping, falling, and tiny gestures. For example, rhythmic oscillations in acceleration data may correspond to walking, whereas abrupt large changes may represent a fall. The naked acceleration signal usually has both gravitational and body motion parts, which are usually separated in preprocessing to exclude the movement-specific acceleration.
ii. ***Gyroscopes***: Gyroscope measures angular velocity or rate of rotation about an axis. Like accelerometers, gyroscopes of HAR systems tend to give information along three orthogonal axes. Whereas accelerometers pick up on linear motion, gyroscopes are required to capture rotational movement, e.g., rotation, torsion, or swinging of limbs. The fusion of accelerometer and gyroscope information offers a more thorough understanding of human movement and better differential diagnosis between actions that may have the same linear acceleration pattern but with different rotations. For instance, running and walking may share similar accelerations, but arm swings and rotations of the body would be clearly recorded by a gyroscope.
iii. ***Magnetometers***: A magnetometer quantifies the direction and magnitude of magnetic fields. Magnetometers are utilized in IMUs to measure absolute orientation against the Earth's north magnetic pole. The data is essential for calibrating the drift that may pile up in the readings of accelerometers and gyroscopes over time, which phenomenon is known as drift. Through supplying a stable reference for the purpose of orientation, magnetometers increase the precision of tracking motion and activity recognition, especially for activities with direction or orientation in space changes. Magnetometers may, however, be sensitive to disturbance by external magnetic fields, a factor that should be taken into consideration at data collection and analysis times.

2.1.3.3 Physiological Sensors

In addition to kinematic information, physiological sensors provide information on the internal responses of the body to activity, giving a richer understanding of human state and effort. Although not measuring movement directly, their data may be strongly correlated with particular activities or states.

i. ***Heart Rate Sensors***: These sensors take the user's heart rate, generally using photoplethysmography (PPG) technology integrated in smartwatches or chest straps. Heart rate information can distinguish the intensity of activity, distinguish resting from exertion, and offer important context for activities that may look alike kinematically but are different in physiological demand (e.g., slow walking compared to fast walking). It is especially useful in fitness tracking, health monitoring, and stress detection.
ii. ***Electromyography (EMG) Sensors***: EMG sensors record the electrical activity generated by skeletal muscles. By being able to detect muscle contractions, EMG can yield direct evidence of muscle activation during an activity. This can be especially helpful in identifying particular gestures, rehabilitation exercises, or activities where small muscle movements are decisive discriminators. Although more invasive than IMUs, EMG provides a distinct view of the biomechanics of human movement.
iii. ***Electroencephalography (EEG) Sensors***: EEG sensors record the brain's electrical activity. Though less typically applied to general body physical activity recognition, EEG can be essential when identifying cognitive actions, mental conditions (e.g., relaxation and concentration), or sleep phases. In advanced HAR applications, like in tracking people with neurological disorders or brain–computer interfaces, EEG information can yield useful additional information.

2.1.3.4 GPS Sensors

Global positioning system (GPS) sensors calculate the device's geographical location. While IMUs are superior at recording subtle body movements, GPS is good at contextualizing the big-picture movements and activities performed outside of buildings. GPS is useful for metrics such as distance traveled, pace, and path, so GPS is good to use for running, cycling, or backpacking. But GPS has limitations, such as high-power requirements and low accuracy in indoor or urban canyon scenarios where the satellite signal is obstructed. So, it is usually combined with other sensors for a better picture of what people are doing, particularly outdoors.

2.1.3.5 Environmental Sensors

Environmental sensors are stationed in a controlled area (e.g., a home, office, or public space) to track the conditions in that area and the presence of human beings, their movement, or interactions with objects within the area. These sensors do not need direct body attachment, thus providing a less invasive approach, and are ideal for ongoing monitoring over long periods in stationary positions.

2.1.3.6 Passive Infrared (PIR) Sensors

PIR sensors respond to infrared radiation changes that are emitted by the heat bodies such as humans. PIR sensors are utilized for presence and motion detection. As a person walks into the sensor's field of view, the infrared pattern change activates the sensor. PIR sensors are low-cost and energy-efficient and make them ubiquitous for use in applications such as automated lighting, security systems, and occupancy detection for smart homes. They will generally only sense movement and are unable to distinguish between various forms of activity or to recognize individuals.

Ultrasonic Sensors

Ultrasonic sensors create high-frequency sound waves and then calculate the time it takes for such waves to bounce off an object and back to the sensor. This enables them to measure the distance of objects and sense movement. For HAR, ultrasonic sensors may be employed for proximity detection, sensing movement within a small area, or even sensing small movements such as breathing. They are less sensitive to lighting levels than vision-based sensors but may be sensitive to environmental conditions such as air currents and can occasionally generate false alarms.

2.1.3.7 Pressure Sensors

Pressure sensors respond to changes in force or pressure. When placed in floors, chairs, beds, or other devices, they can deduce human activities like rising from bed, sitting down, lying in bed, or walking across a room. For example, a floor pressure mat can monitor footsteps and gait patterns, while pressure sensors in a chair can signal sitting time or changes in posture. These sensors do not intrude and can supply useful contextual information regarding activities executed in particular places.

2.1.3.8 Ambient Light Sensors

Ambient light sensors quantify the ambient intensity of light within an environment. Although they do not measure human activity directly, variations in ambient light can offer contextual information to support activity identification. As an example, an abrupt reduction in light levels can signify that an individual has extinguished the lights when retiring to bed, or an increase can imply that they have opened window curtains. Such contextual information can be used to disambiguate actions that would otherwise be hard to identify through motion data alone.

2.1.3.9 Sound Sensors (Microphones)

Microphones, or acoustic sensors, receive sound signals from the surroundings. They may hold precious information regarding human activities like footsteps, speech, coughing, object manipulation (e.g., door opening and washing dishes), or even the sounds made when particular exercises are performed. Sophisticated audio processing methods like speech recognition and sound event detection can be used to extract features of these audio streams for HAR. Nevertheless, privacy issues and the occurrence of background noise are main obstacles while utilizing microphones for HAR.

2.1.3.10 Temperature Sensors

Temperature sensors detect the ambient temperature of an area. Like ambient light sensors, temperature information mostly gives context about the environment. Yet, variations in local temperature will on occasion suggest the presence of people (e.g., body heat influencing a nearby sensor) or activity that produces heat (e.g., cooking). Though it is not a main sensor for explicit activity detection, temperature information may add to a fuller view of the environment and human interaction therein.

2.1.4 Vision-Based Sensors

Vision-based sensors, mostly cameras, record visual data of body movement and interaction. Although the spotlight in this journal is on "all sensors," and the initial question highlighted non-vision sensors, it is significant to briefly take note of the large contribution of vision-based methods to HAR. These systems interpret streams of video to detect activities, usually utilizing methods such as pose estimation, action recognition, and body part tracking.

2.1.4.1 Cameras

i. ***RGB Cameras***: Conventional color cameras capture visual data, which can be processed by computer vision algorithms to identify and classify human activities. They are used quite routinely for surveillance, gesture recognition, sports analytics, and many other applications. Yet, their performance is strongly sensitive to illumination, occlusions, and privacy requirements.
ii. ***Depth Cameras***: These (e.g., Microsoft Kinect, Intel RealSense) capture 3D spatial data and, in addition to color images, yield a depth map. This enables stronger pose estimation and activity recognition since they are less affected by lighting changes and can better distinguish foreground from background. Depth

data is especially helpful in distinguishing activities involving subtle movement or changes in body posture.

iii. ***Thermal Cameras***: Thermal cameras pick up infrared radiation released by objects, so they are able to "see" heat signatures. They can be beneficial in low-light environments or privacy issues, as they do not record identifiable facial features. Thermal imaging can pick up human presence and movement and under certain circumstances distinguish between activities based on heat signatures created through exertion.

Although strong, vision-based HAR systems can be plagued by issues of privacy, computational expense, and environmental sensitivity. They tend to be supplemented by other sensor modalities to mitigate these shortcomings.

2.1.5 Hybrid Sensor Systems

Hybrid sensor systems fuse information from various types of sensors and tend to mix wearable, environmental, and sometimes vision-based modalities. The theory underlying hybrid systems is to take advantage of the strengths of each type of sensor while compensating for their respective weaknesses. For example, merging data from an IMU sensor on a smartwatch with pressure sensor data on a smart floor can yield a more precise and detailed description of walking, sitting, and falling activities. Data fusion algorithms are used to integrate the heterogeneous streams of data, generating better accuracy, robustness, and context awareness in HAR. The multimodal strategy makes it possible to have a richer representation of human activity, facilitating the identification of more sophisticated and subtle behavior that may be hard to identify with one sensor modality.

2.1.6 Data Preprocessing

Raw sensor data, no matter the source, is seldom directly in a format conducive to machine learning algorithms. They are usually beset by noise, inconsistencies, and redundancy that can be detrimental to the functioning of HAR models. Data preprocessing is an essential step in the HAR pipeline that converts raw sensor signals into a clean, consistent, and informative form. This process entails some key steps.

2.1.6.1 Noise Filtering

Sensor data is prone to all kinds of noise, which may be caused by sensor imperfections, environmental noise, or accidental human movements. Noise filtering tries to eliminate such unwanted signals while retaining the activity-related information. Some typical filtering methods are as follows:

i. ***Low-pass filters***: Low-pass filters permit low-frequency signals (slow, deliberate movements) to pass through while suppressing high-frequency noise (e.g., sensor jitter, abrupt shocks). A Butterworth low-pass filter, for example, is frequently employed to isolate the gravitational component from the body acceleration component of accelerometer data.
ii. ***High-pass filters***: In contrast, high-pass filters permit high-frequency signals to pass through, which can be beneficial in isolating quick movements or transient events.
iii. ***Band-pass filters***: These integrate features of both the low-pass and the high-pass filters, which enable signals in a certain frequency range to pass through, isolating activity-specific frequencies in effect.
iv. ***Median filters***: Nonlinear filters that are efficient at eliminating salt-and-pepper noise or abrupt spikes in the data without smearing edges, advantageous for conserving sharp transitions in activity data.

The selection of filtering approach varies based on the kind of sensor, the nature of the noise, and the nature of the activities to be recognized.

2.1.6.2 Segmentation (Windowing)

Human activity is ongoing in nature, whereas machine learning models usually have to work with discrete, fixed-size input samples. Segmentation, or windowing, is the process of breaking the ongoing stream of sensor measurements into smaller, manageable pieces or windows. The windows are then processed individually as one sample per window for activity classification. There are two main segmentation approaches:

i. **Fixed-size sliding windows**: The most popular approach, in which data is separated into fixed-sized windows (e.g., 2.56 s) of a specified length with a specified overlap (e.g., 50%). The overlap guarantees that actions falling at the ends of windows are not lost and offer additional training examples. The size of the window is important; a window that is too small may fail to encompass the complete dynamics of an activity, while one too big may conflate a number of activities in one segment.
ii. **Activity-defined windows**: Sometimes activities can be partitioned according to particular events or transitions, for example, the beginning and finishing of a movement cycle. This method demands more advanced event detection algorithms but can result in more accurate activity boundaries.

2.1.6.3 Feature Extraction

Feature extraction is the extraction of a set of informative, discriminative features from the raw or preprocessed sensor data for each segment. These features should represent the key properties of an activity in a compact and efficient form to make it easier for machine learning models to be able to differentiate between activities. Features can be generally classified into time-domain and frequency-domain features:

a. **Time-Domain Features**: These are computed directly from the raw time-series data over a window. Typical time-domain features include:

    i. **Mean**: Central tendency of the sensor signal, which is the average value of the sensor signal.
    ii. **Standard Deviation**: Quantifies the spread of data points around the mean, which denotes the variability of the signal.
    iii. **Variance**: The square of the standard deviation.
    iv. **Root Mean Square (RMS)**: The amplitude of the signal, used for expressing overall activity level.
    v. **Min/Max Values**: The window's minimum and maximum values, expressing the extent of the signal.
    vi. **Skewness**: Quantifies the asymmetry of the data distribution.
    vii. **Kurtosis**: Quantifies the peakedness or flatness of the data distribution.
    viii. **Correlation**: Quantifies the correlation between signals from varying sensor axes or different sensors.

b. **Frequency-Domain Features**: These are obtained by converting the signal in the time domain to the frequency domain, generally by methods such as the fast Fourier transform (FFT). Frequency-domain features unveil periodic components and most prominent frequencies in the signal, which tend to be strongly typical of particular activities. Some examples are as follows:

    i. **Energy of Frequency Components**: The power or energy within particular frequency bands.
    ii. **Dominant Frequencies**: The most powerful frequencies, which represent the main rhythmic patterns of an activity.
    iii. **Spectral Entropy**: Quantifies the predictability or randomness of the signal in the frequency domain.

For multi-sensor systems, features are frequently extracted from each sensor separately and then combined to create an integrated feature vector. The choice of suitable features is important for the performance of HAR models because well-designed features can greatly ease the learning process.

2.1.7 Feature Selection and Dimensionality Reduction

Upon feature extraction, the derived feature vector is usually highly dimensional, comprising irrelevant or redundant features. High dimensionality contributes to higher computational cost, overfitting, and less model generalization. Techniques of feature selection and dimensionality reduction are used to reduce these problems:

a. **Feature Selection**: Choosing a subset of the most significant features from the initial group. Techniques encompass filter methods (e.g., correlation-based feature selection), wrapper methods (e.g., recursive feature elimination), and embedded methods (e.g., Lasso regularization). The aim is to learn features that are highly discriminatory for various activities.
b. **Dimensionality Reduction**: These methods map the high-dimensional feature space into a lower-dimensional space with as much of the original information as possible. Some popular methods are as follows:

    i. **Principal Component Analysis (PCA)**: A linear transformation method that determines the principal components (directions of maximum variance) in the data and maps the data onto a lower-dimensional subspace spanned by these components.
    ii. **t-Distributed Stochastic Neighbor Embedding (t-SNE)**: A nonlinear dimensionality reduction method well-adapted for visualizing data of high dimension by projecting it onto a 2D or 3D space, in the process maintaining local neighborhoods.

Feature selection and dimensionality reduction both assist in enhancing model efficiency, saving training time, and increasing the interpretability of the models.

2.1.7.1 Data Normalization and Imputation

a. **Normalization**: The sensor data can differ drastically in scale and range from one sensor, person, or even one recording session to another. Normalization (or standardization) ranges the feature values to a comparable scale (e.g., 0–1) or normalizes them to have a zero mean and unit variance. This avoids features with larger numerical scales from taking over the learning process and enables machine learning algorithms to learn faster and better. Popular normalization methods are min–max scaling and *Z*-score standardization.
b. **Missing Value Imputation**: In the course of data acquisition, sensor values can occasionally be missing because of faulty sensors, errors in transmission, or temporary loss of connection. Missing data has the potential to significantly impair the performance of HAR models. Imputation methods are employed to estimate and complete the missing data points. Basic imputation techniques involve filling in the missing values with the mean, median, or mode of the feature. Advanced methods may employ interpolation, regression, or machine learning algorithms to estimate the missing values based on the available data.

The right treatment of the missing values is essential to keep data intact and make the HAR system robust.

2.1.8 Internet of Things as Enabling Technology in HAR and Health Care

In last few years a lot of advancements have taken place in sensor networks and smart and intelligent devices. As a result, a revolution has taken place in diverse fields like defense, online gaming, sports, and especially health care, to mention a few. World Health Organization (WHO) published a report few years ago that number of senior citizens is increasing all over the world [1]. US Bureau of the Census also generated similar reports which tells that the number of old people is expected to be doubled by 2025 [1]. Lifestyle changes have led to an increase in cardiovascular problems, obesity, and other chronic diseases. Healthcare expenditure is also increasing by leaps and bounds. This is leading to a decline in the quality of services in the overloaded healthcare system. Use of information and communication technology (ICT) in healthcare system must be increased, and it is absolutely necessary at this critical juncture of time. It provides higher quality of healthcare services. It can be used to provide telemedicine too. Telemedicine combines telecommunication and information technology to provide remote health care including remote diagnosis and treatment of patients. It opens a new dimension in modern-day medical science. In sensor-based health monitoring, wearable or implantable sensors are attached to human body for getting physiological information from the patients. This technique is called wireless body area network or WBAN [2]. Sensed health vitals are sent to coordinator device, mostly smart phone or laptop, supporting user mobility through short-range communication such as WiFi and Bluetooth. Data then further gets transmitted to cloud-based medical server from coordinator device through access point over the Internet. Analysis of the data in the server leads to knowledge about required health care for the corresponding person. Sensor-based monitoring of health without direct intervention of human is the main objective of this entire process. However, this method can be used if sensor-based devices are comfortable and also easy to use. Data collected in server will be analyzed, and if any abnormality is detected, appropriate measures can be taken immediately, otherwise that may cause havoc in the patients' life. Standard for WBAN has been defined in IEEE 802.15.6 with data transmission rate in the range of 75.9 kbps–15.6 Mbps. WBAN interacts with Internet and Bluetooth, ZigBee, WPAN, as well. WBAN can support up to 256 nodes. Sensor nodes should be able to transmit at 0.1 mW with the maximum being not more than 1 mW [5–7]. WBAN monitors human physical conditions and transfers 2 data to a central node via wireless channel as shown in Fig. 2.1. WBAN and smartphone sensors are very often utilized for HAR and monitoring purposes [8].

Since this health information is sent through insecure channel, data suffers from lack of privacy. Adversary can apply different security attacks like man-in-the-middle attack, replay attack, impersonation attack, modification attack, etc. [3], to

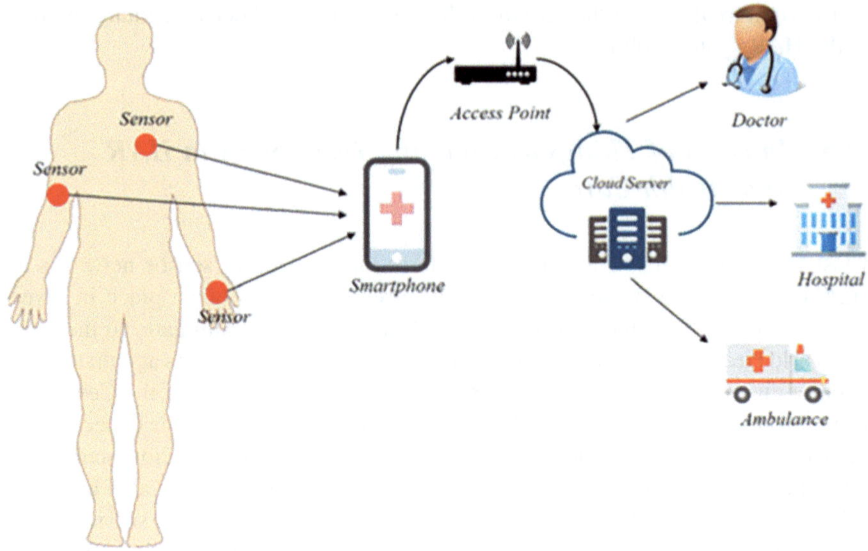

Fig. 2.1 Smart healthcare framework

gather private information of the patient or can alter the information. If adversary alters the vital health information, doctor will provide advice based on altered data which can be life threatening. Hence, the security of the patient-related information is a prime concern. Security can be ensured by applying traditional cryptographic techniques to achieve the confidentiality and integrity of the data as well as intrusion detection technique can help the network administrator to detect various cyber-attacks and act accordingly.

2.1.9 Machine Learning in HAR

The healthcare industry has been significantly transformed by implementing machine learning techniques, providing novel and advanced approaches to address intricate challenges. These methodologies enhance the quality of patient care, optimize operational efficiency, and facilitate advancements in medical research. The machine learning (ML) techniques can be broadly categorized into three types, namely:

Supervised Learning

In supervised learning, data inputs and their desired outputs are utilized for training a program to map new data inputs. Supervised learning may be divided into two categories—classification, that deals with discrete output and regression, which predicts continuous outcome [9]. In both the cases, the system is trained with existing data, and then, the learned system is used to predict the outcome on new data.

Regression analysis is a powerful statistical tool for forecasting real values, such as accelerometer readings. Depending on the nature of the independent variable, it can predict future values or unveil unknown present ones. The spectrum of regression techniques spans from straightforward linear regression to more advanced methods like support vector regression (SVR) and random forests regression [10]. These models enable us to uncover meaningful relationships within data and make informed predictions, facilitating decision-making across various fields, from finance to science and beyond.

Classification is a crucial data analysis technique, enabling the prediction discrete groups rather than continuous values. It finds application across diverse fields, such as medicine and business. Various classification methods are available, each suited to different data types and complexities. Linear models like logistic regression and support vector machines excel at straightforward separations. Conversely, nonlinear approaches handle intricate relationships and patterns, including K-nearest neighbors (K-NN), kernel SVM, and random forests [11]. These models empower data scientists to enhance decision-making, whether diagnosing diseases or targeting specific customer segments, thereby bolstering numerous domains with improved insights. The following classification-based algorithms are particularly popular in healthcare domain.

Support Vector Machine (SVM)

Support vector machine (SVM) algorithms are invaluable in healthcare data analysis due to their computational prowess, catering to various clinical objectives. SVM tackles regression, classification, and outlier detection, effectively identifying ailments like cancer, hypertension, and diabetes. In binary classification, SVM utilizes hyperplanes, separating data points efficiently. For multiclass scenarios, it employs one-to-one or one-to-rest strategies. In healthcare applications, SVM excels in breast cancer diagnosis by classifying mammography data and predicting diabetes through factors like body mass index and blood glucose levels [12]. Its interpretability and accuracy make it suitable for linear and nonlinear data, improving predictive accuracy. However, it faces challenges with large datasets due to extended training times and may struggle when target classes overlap, necessitating careful parameter tuning [13]. In the SVM classification formula, the decision boundary is defined as

$$f(x) = \sin(WX + b)$$

Logistic Regression

Logistic regression is a statistical technique for predicting categorical outcomes based on several independent variables. In smart healthcare systems, it plays a pivotal role in detecting diseases like breast cancer [14]. In health care, logistic regression is also used to predict outcomes for patients, like how likely it is that a patient will need to be readmitted or how likely it is that they will have problems after surgery. This helps make choices about treatment and how to use resources.

K-Nearest Neighbors (KNN)

The K-nearest neighbor (KNN) algorithm is a prominent instance-based learning method that holds significance in the healthcare domain. In this approach, instances are characterized by n attribute-value pairs, and it retrieves a set of relevant instances from memory to classify new queries. Its appeal lies in its straightforwardness and capacity to function effectively with limited data. The fundamental aspect of KNN involves the computation of distances, with the Euclidean distance often employed in the n-dimensional space. In health care, KNN can predict patient outcomes based on similar medical histories [15]. For instance, it can help identify personalized treatment plans by finding the nearest neighbors (patients with similar health profiles) for a given case, offering tailored medical recommendations.

Naive Bayes

Naive Bayes is a versatile classification algorithm that performs exceptionally well in binary and multiclass categorization, especially with categorical input variables. In health care, Naive Bayes is valuable for predicting diseases based on symptoms due to its efficient handling of nonnumerical data. For instance, given symptom probabilities, it calculates the likelihood of a disease's presence [16]. For example, Naive Bayes can rank conditions in a symptom dataset by their possibility, aiding timely diagnoses.

Decision Tree

The decision tree (DT) algorithm is a versatile tool for classification and regression, offering solutions in a tree-like structure that clarifies decision processes. This representation is explicit and visual, with internal nodes representing attributes and leaf nodes containing class labels. It operates on if–then rules, allowing for easy comprehension. In health care, DT proves invaluable. In medical diagnosis, for instance, the algorithm can determine the possibility that a patient has a particular condition based on symptoms and test results [17]. Mathematically, the algorithm uses recursive partitioning to find the best attribute to split the data at each node, often employing impurity measures like Gini impurity or entropy: Pruning is crucial to enhance performance and reduce complexity. It eliminates branches of low importance, improving the model's generalization. In health care, a decision tree (DT) can guide treatment decisions based on patient characteristics [18], optimizing care pathways and resource allocation.

Random Forest Classification

Random forest (RF) is a powerful predictive machine learning model that leverages ensemble learning. It combines multiple decision trees to enhance prediction accuracy. The key idea is that uncorrelated models, represented by individual decision trees, perform better collectively. For instance, in medical diagnosis, RF can integrate diverse patient data (symptoms and demographics) and individual decision tree (DT) to enhance disease prediction [19]. Each tree contributes a vote, and the most voted diagnosis becomes the final prediction. The low correlation between decision trees reduces errors, ensuring a more accurate overall outcome in healthcare applications.

2.1.10 Unsupervised Machine Learning

Unsupervised learning operates on unlabeled datasets, making it ideal for discovering hidden data patterns. Without predefined labels, it is valuable when data characteristics are unclear.

Clustering, an essential technique, groups similar data based on inherent similarities. In health care, unsupervised learning aids in patient segmentation for personalized treatments or identifying disease subtypes within large patient populations, improving precision medicine [20]. For instance, it can classify patients with similar symptoms into distinct groups, leading to more tailored healthcare interventions.

- **K-means clustering**

One widely used clustering algorithm is K-means. In K-means clustering, centroids are updated, and data point assignments change iteratively until clusters stabilize. In health care, K-means can segment patient populations based on similar health metrics [21], helping hospitals customize treatment plans and allocate resources effectively as patient data evolves.

DBSCAN

Another algorithm, density-based spatial clustering of applications with noise (DBSCAN), is an unsupervised clustering technique beneficial for automatically determining cluster numbers and handling arbitrarily shaped clusters.

In health care, DBSCAN plays a pivotal role in patient data analysis. For instance, it can identify dense regions of patients with similar health profiles, aiding in cohort discovery. Patients with MinPts (a minimum number of shared health characteristics) are considered core patients, while those directly linked to them are border patients. This helps segment patients into meaningful clusters, such as identifying patients with similar disease progressions for tailored treatments. DBSCAN can also detect outlier patients, which is valuable for flagging unusual health records or potential anomalies in medical data [22]. This clustering approach effectively manages high-density and low-density patient clusters, enhancing healthcare analytics and decision-making. A few more popular unsupervised algorithms used in smart health care are mentioned below.

Hierarchical Clustering

It is a powerful technique that effectively aids disease taxonomy by forming a hierarchical tree of clusters. Grouping-related conditions based on symptom similarity [23] is an indispensable tool for identifying interrelated diseases. Principal component analysis (PCA): PCA reduces high-dimensional healthcare data while retaining essential information. It aids in visualizing and understanding patient data [24], allowing for better diagnostics.

Autoencoders

These neural networks are employed for feature learning and dimensionality reduction [25] in medical image analysis. They have been used for anomaly detection in X-ray images to identify fractures.

Gaussian Mixture Models (GMM): GMM assumes that data is generated from a mixture of Gaussian distributions. It is utilized to model patient data for segmentation [26], e.g., classifying EEG signals to diagnose epilepsy.

The literature discussed above explained different approaches for developing innovative healthcare devices. This helped us to identify areas where we can improve our proposed designs. We found that more work needs to be done to keep senior citizens' cost and convenience in mind. Models based on real data and with proper clinical support are also relatively rare. Many works rely on storing and analyzing systems that depend on cloud-based processing. Support for hybrid architecture using machine learning (ML) and threshold-based (TB) methods is occasional. State-of-the-art processing at the IoT level by Raspberry Pi or similar devices is also rare. Not many researchers are interested in heterogeneous sensor-based work on physical devices due to the complexity involved. Using a smartphone as a sensor hub is widespread, but its implementation in real-world cases is rare. This aspect inspired us to develop our first smartphone-based fall detection system implemented on real-life Parkinson's disease (PD) patients to reduce their fear of falling (FoF). The next chapter will introduce this system in more detail.

2.1.11 Deep Learning-Based Methods

Deep learning as a machine learning method and artificial intelligence techniques for feature extraction has come a long way since its resurgence in 2006. The upsurge in deep learning research is fueled by its ability to extract salient features from raw sensor data without relying on laboriously handcrafted features [13, 20]. Furthermore, in the area of human activity recognition, for instance, complex human activities are translational invariant and hierarchical in nature, and the same activities can be performed in different ways by the same participants. In some cases, activities can be a starting point for other complex activities; running and jogging might not be distinguishable depending on the age and health condition for the person performing the activity. Deep learning [27] is a machine learning technique that uses representational learning to discover feature representation in raw sensor data automatically, unlike classical machine learning (support vector machine, k-nearest neighbor, K-means, etc.) that require a human engineered feature to perform optimally. Over the years, deep learning has provided extensive applications in image recognition speech recognition, medicine and pharmacy, natural language processing, and recently in human activity recognition. Extensive number of deep learning methods have been proposed recently, and these methods can be broadly classified into restricted Boltzmann machine, deep autoencoder, sparse coding, convolutional neural network, recurrent neural networks, etc. [28, 29]. Some of these methods are reviewed in the section below, outlining the characteristics, advantages, and drawbacks of each method.

Deep learning, as we have knew just before that this is an offshoot of machine learning based on the brain structure and operation, has transformed numerous applications of artificial intelligence, including human activity recognition. Deep learning architectures, especially convolutional neural networks (CNNs) and recurrent neural networks (RNNs), have shown better performance in HAR [30, 31] by learning hierarchical features automatically from raw or lightly preprocessed sensor data, lessening manual feature engineering.

Some of the methods are briefly described below just for readers' ready reference.

2.1.11.1 Convolutional Neural Networks (CNN)

Convolutional neural networks (CNNs), which were initially designed for image processing, have been found to be extremely useful in HAR, particularly when used with sensor data that can either be viewed as one-dimensional signals or converted into two-dimensional representations (such as spectrograms). CNNs are particularly good at detecting local structures and spatial hierarchies of data using convolutional layers. In HAR, these layers can be trained to recognize particular patterns of movement (e.g., an acceleration peak for a step) irrespective of their location in the sensor window. Pooling layers then lower the dimensionality of features that have been learned, making the model less sensitive to small changes. The major benefits of CNNs in HAR are that they can automatically extract the features of interest, are insensitive to variations in the placement of sensors, and can process vast amounts of data [32, 33]. They are particularly useful for detecting activities with clear, repetitive patterns.

2.1.11.2 Recurrent Neural Networks (RNN)

Recurrent neural networks (RNNs) are specially developed to handle sequential data and thus are naturally appropriate for time-series sensor data in HAR. In contrast to feedforward neural networks, RNNs possess internal memory that enables them to keep track of past time step information, allowing them to learn temporal dependencies and contextual cues essential for activity recognition [34]. But the classic RNNs are plagued by the vanishing gradient issue, which restricts them from learning long-term dependencies. To solve this, special RNN architectures have been proposed.

2.1.11.3 Long Short-Term Memory (LSTM) Networks

LSTMs are a variant of RNNs that mitigate the vanishing gradient issue by introducing "gates" (input, forget, and output gates) that control the information flow in and out of the cell state. This gating mechanism enables LSTMs to selectively forget or remember information along long sequences, enabling them to be excellent at modeling complicated temporal relationships in HAR data. LSTMs are especially strong at detecting activities that consist of complicated sequences of movements or activities that last for longer durations, such as walking upstairs or doing a sequence of exercises.

2.1.11.4 Gated Recurrent Units (GRUs)

GRUs are a lightweight alternative to LSTMs, putting the forget and input gates together into an "update gate" and combining the cell state and hidden state. Although less complex in structure, GRUs tend to learn just as well as LSTMs using fewer parameters, resulting in more efficient training times and lower computational requirements. Like LSTMs, GRUs are excellent at capturing long-term dependencies in sequential sensor data, making them a strong choice for various HAR tasks.

2.1.11.5 Edge Computing in HAR

Edge computing has emerged as a transformative paradigm for human activity recognition (HAR), addressing the critical challenges of latency, privacy, and resource constraints inherent in traditional cloud-based approaches. This distributed computing framework brings data processing closer to the source, enabling real-time activity recognition on resource-constrained devices while preserving user privacy and reducing bandwidth consumption [35].

2.1.12 Key Advantages of Using Edge Computing in HAR

There are various advantages of using edge computing in human activity recognition. These are described as below:

Low Latency and Real-Time Detection

Edge computing significantly reduces latency by processing data locally rather than transmitting it to distant cloud servers. Traditional cloud-based HARsystems suffer from high latency due to the round-trip communication between edge devices and centralized servers, which can be particularly problematic for real-time applications [36]. By moving computation to the edge, systems can achieve near-instantaneous decision-making, with inference times as low as 21 ms on microcontrollers.

Privacy-Aware and Energy-Efficient Computing

The raw sensor data along with identity-related data of the user is confined to the user-specific edge device, and data processing in limited to the edge device thus avoids the need to transmit data to the remote cloud server over the open wireless links. This ensures user data privacy and user identity privacy.

This causes less energy consumption and delay in data processing.

Edge AI Frameworks and Tools Used

TensorFlow Lite/LiteRT: Google's LiteRT (formerly TensorFlow Lite) has become a cornerstone technology for deploying HAR models on edge devices. It provides optimized runtime for on-device AI with support for quantization and hardware acceleration.

Edge Impulse Platform: This platform facilitates the deployment of lightweight models on microcontrollers, enabling real-time HAR with minimal resource consumption.

Federated Learning Approaches: Federated learning frameworks enable collaborative model training across distributed edge devices while preserving data privacy. These systems allow distributed edge devices while preserving data privacy. These systems allow personalized HAR models without centralizing sensitive data.

Edge computing represents a paradigm shift in human activity recognition, offering significant advantages in terms of latency, privacy, and resource efficiency. The combination of lightweight deep learning models, advanced optimization techniques, and distributed computing architectures enables real-time HAR on resource-constrained devices. While challenges remain in areas such as model management and connectivity, ongoing research and technological advances continue to expand the capabilities and applications of edge-based HAR systems. The field is rapidly evolving, with new architectures, optimization techniques, and applications emerging regularly. As edge computing hardware becomes more capable and affordable, we can expect to see even more sophisticated HAR systems deployed across various domains, from health care and smart homes to industrial automation and beyond. The key to success will be continued innovation in model efficiency, system optimization, and cross-platform compatibility, ensuring that the benefits of edge-based HAR can be realized across diverse use cases and deployment scenarios.

2.1.13 Cloud Computing in HAR

The rapid advancement in data science, sensors, IoT, 5G communications with high bandwidth, multimodal sensors, and devices generating complex and huge data has emerged with a need of cloud servers in the late nineteenth century for mainly storage purpose and then as different resource pool also in the form SaaS, PaaS, and IaaS. Complex and intelligent models such as machine learning, deep learning, artificial intelligence, and neural network run at cloud on huge datasets to generate patterns. Thus, it has become very much feasible to design and develop various real-life applications coining on the facilities provided by the cloud computing.

One of the most emerging applications of cloud computing is in health care. Recently, various physicians and healthcare practitioners around the world have explored cloud health care in developing a strong, consistent, and economical cloud program-based design to deal with a greater number of simultaneous requirements from global healthcare facilities.

Cloud computing has become a fundamental enabling technology in the field of human activity recognition (HAR), revolutionizing how large amounts of sensor and video data are processed, analyzed, and stored for real-world applications. Here is an overview of its role and advantages:

Important Roles of Cloud Computing in HAR

Cloud is reliable enabler of huge data processing and storage. Cloud setup provides virtually unlimited storage and computing resources. Hence, massive sensory raw data collected from different heterogeneous sensors in different format could efficiently be stored and analyzed and processed using several AI-based complex models [31].

Deployment of Complex Models

Because HAR often relies on deep learning algorithms that demand significant computing power (especially during training), cloud computing enables the use of sophisticated models (e.g., hybrid CNN-LSTM and CNN-GRU architectures) that would be too computationally intensive for edge devices. The cloud environment supports high-accuracy recognition by providing on-demand GPU/TPU acceleration for model training and inference.

Benefits of Processing HAR Multimodal Data at Cloud

- Enhance accuracy in recognition of activity
- Resource utilization could be ensured in efficient manner
- Scalable and flexible
- Privacy-aware solutions.

2.2 Conclusion

Human activity recognition and fall detection using sensors, IoT, and cloud with application of machine learning and deep learning models are an immensely popular domain of research. Work in this domain is not limited to research only but also are being used in real life for enhancing quality living. HAR and FD need support of different enabling technologies for smooth and efficient functioning of this huge heterogeneous sensory data-based recognition that demands real-time performance. This chapter highlights all the small details of these enabling technologies and their role in HAR.

References

1. Thakur, D., & Biswas, S. (2020). Smartphone based human activity monitoring and recognition using ML and DL: A comprehensive survey. *Journal of Ambient Intelligence and Humanized Computing, 11*(11), 5433–5444.
2. Zhang, Y., et al. (2023). Automatic detection system for velopharyngeal insufficiency based on acoustic signals from nasal and oral channels. *Diagnostics, 13*(16), 2714.
3. Yuan, K., et al. (2023). Smartphone-based hand-held polarized light microscope for on-site pharmaceutical crystallinity characterization. *Analytical and Bioanalytical Chemistry,* 1–10.
4. https://www.who.int/news-room/fact-sheets/detail/ageing-and-health
5. Kumar, P., Chauhan, S., & Awasthi, L. K. (2024). Human activity recognition (HAR) using deep learning: Review, methodologies, progress and future research directions. *Archives of Computational Methods in Engineering, 31*(1), 179–219.
6. Fu, B., et al. (2020). Sensing technology for human activity recognition: A comprehensive survey. *IEEE Access, 8*, 83791–83820.
7. Contoli, C., Freschi, V., & Lattanzi, E. (2024). Energy-aware human activity recognition for wearable devices: A comprehensive review. *Pervasive and Mobile Computing, 104*, 101976.
8. Lara, O. D., & Labrador, M. A. (2012). A survey on human activity recognition using wearable sensors. *IEEE Communications Surveys & Tutorials, 15*(3), 1192–1209.
9. De-La-Hoz-Franco, E., et al. (2018). Sensor-based datasets for human activity recognition—A systematic review of literature. *IEEE Access, 6*, 59192–59210.
10. Mehmood, K., Imran, H. A., & Latif, U. (2020). HARDenseNet: A 1D DenseNet inspired convolutional neural network for human activity recognition with inertial sensors. In *2020 IEEE 23rd International Multitopic Conference (INMIC)*. IEEE.
11. Mishra, R., et al. (2024). Optimizing activity recognition through dominant axis identification in inertial sensors. *IEEE Sensors Letters*.
12. Rezaei, A., et al. (2022). An unobtrusive human activity recognition system using low resolution thermal sensors, machine and deep learning. *IEEE Transactions on Biomedical Engineering, 70*(1), 115–124.
13. FFT spectrum spread with machine learning (ML) analysis of triaxial acceleration from shirt pocket and torso for sensing coughs while walking.
14. Wang, Z., et al. (2023). Recognition of approximate motions of human based on micro-Doppler features. *IEEE Sensors Journal, 23*(11), 12388–12397.
15. Sassi, M., et al. (2024). Classification of shoulder rehabilitation exercises by using wearable systems and machine learning algorithms. *IEEE Sensors Journal, 24*(14), 22934–22944.
16. Tabrizi, S. S., Pashazadeh, S., & Javani, V. (2020). Comparative study of table tennis forehand strokes classification using deep learning and SVM. *IEEE Sensors Journal, 20*(22), 13552–13561.
17. Ehrnsperger, M. G., et al. (2020). Real-time gesture detection based on machine learning classification of continuous wave radar signals. *IEEE Sensors Journal, 21*(6), 8310–8322.
18. Nalwaya, A., Das, K., & Pachori, R. B. (2024). An automated framework for human emotion detection from multichannel EEG signals. *IEEE Sensors Journal, 24*(13), 20920–20927.
19. Thakur, D., & Biswas, S. (2021). Feature fusion using deep learning for smartphone based human activity recognition. *International Journal of Information Technology, 13*(4), 1615–1624.
20. Ankalaki, S. (2024). Simple to complex, single to concurrent sensor-based human activity recognition: Perception and open challenges. *IEEE Access, 12*, 93450–93486.

21. Zhang, L., et al. (2024). A multi-channel hybrid deep learning framework for multi-sensor fusion enabled human activity recognition. *Alexandria Engineering Journal, 91*, 472–485.
22. Athota, R. K., & Sumathi, D. (2022). Human activity recognition based on hybrid learning algorithm for wearable sensor data. *Measurement: Sensors, 24*, 100512.
23. Ghate, V., & Hemalatha, C. S. (2023). A comprehensive comparison of machine learning approaches with hyper-parameter tuning for smartphone sensor-based human activity recognition. *Measurement: Sensors, 30*, 100925.
24. Garcia-Gonzalez, D., et al. (2023). New machine learning approaches for real-life human activity recognition using smartphone sensor-based data. *Knowledge-Based Systems, 262*, 110260.
25. Imanzadeh, S., Tanha, J., & Jalili, M. (2024). Ensemble of deep learning techniques to human activity recognition using smart phone signals. *Multimedia Tools and Applications, 83*(42), 89635–89664.
26. Choudhury, N. A., & Soni, B. (2024). In-depth analysis of design & development for sensor-based human activity recognition system. *Multimedia Tools and Applications, 83*(29), 73233–73272.
27. Mallik, M., Sarkar, G., & Chowdhury, C. (2024). A deep learning framework for smartphone based human activity recognition. *Mobile Networks and Applications, 29*(1), 29–41.
28. Mittal, P. (2022). Machine learning (ML) based human activity recognition model using smart sensors in IoT environment. In *2022 12th International Conference on Cloud Computing, Data Science & Engineering (confluence)*. IEEE.
29. Mani, N., Haridoss, P., & George, B. (2023). Evaluation of a combined conductive fabric-based suspender system and machine learning approach for human activity recognition. *IEEE Open Journal of Instrumentation and Measurement, 2*, 1–10.
30. Raziani, S., & Azimbagirad, M. (2022). Deep CNN hyperparameter optimization algorithms for sensor-based human activity recognition. *Neuroscience Informatics, 2*(3), 100078.
31. Gupta, S. (2021). Deep learning based human activity recognition (HAR) using wearable sensor data. *International Journal of Information Management Data Insights, 1*(2), 100046.
32. Saidani, O., et al. (2023). An efficient human activity recognition using hybrid features and transformer model. *IEEE Access, 11*, 101373–101386.
33. Uddin, M. A., et al. (2024). Deep learning-based human activity recognition using CNN, ConvLSTM, and LRCN. *International Journal of Cognitive Computing in Engineering, 5*, 259–268.
34. Duan, H., et al. (2024). Wearable-based behaviour interpolation for semi-supervised human activity recognition. *Information Sciences, 665*, 120393.
35. Wazwaz, A. A., Amin, K. M., Semari, N. A., & Ghanem, T. F. (2023). Enhancing human activity recognition using features reduction in IoT edge and Azure cloud. *Decision Analytics Journal, 8*, 100282.
36. Biswas, S., & Chowdhury, C. (2020, October). Smartphone and sensor based health monitoring enabled with IoT and ML. In *22nd International Conference on Human-Computer Interaction with Mobile Devices and Services* (pp. 1–3).

Chapter 3
Machine Learning in Human Activity Recognition

3.1 Introduction

In today's world, there are more older people who live alone and often have chronic illnesses that can be prevented by keeping an eye on their daily activities [1]. However, using lots of sensors you wear on your body [2] can be bothersome for these elderly people [3]. But now, there is a better way to monitor them without causing any inconvenience. We have smart devices like smartphones [4, 5] and smartwatches that can help. These gadgets are like tiny computers you can carry with you. Sensors embedded in smart handheld [6] devices can be incredibly valuable in gathering information about people's activities and behaviors. Most people carry smartphones [7] with them almost all the time. These smartphones come equipped with a variety of built-in sensors like accelerometers, gyroscopes, compasses, proximity sensors, light sensors, and GPS [8, 9]. These sensors can collect data related to users' activities. Moreover, smartphones can transmit this data wirelessly via interfaces such as Wi-Fi or 3G/4G to a nursing station or a medical server. They can keep an eye on things like your heart rate and figure out how you are sitting or moving. They can even tell if something strange is happening. All this information goes to the people who take care of these elderly folks or their doctors. This helps the caregivers or doctors understand what is going on with the older person's health without needing to visit them in person [3]. It makes it easier to spot problems and treat diseases correctly.

These triaxial accelerometers [10, 11] and gyroscope sensors enable the smartphone to detect and record the user's movements and posture, offering insights into their physical activities. Additionally, the smartphone utilizes Wi-Fi technology for location identification, allowing it to determine the user's whereabouts by analyzing nearby Wi-Fi access points. Meanwhile, a Bluetooth-enabled smart band and fitness tracker work in tandem to track the user's heart rate and count their steps throughout the day. This real-time data on heart rate and step count helps in assessing the user's cardiovascular health and activity level. Furthermore, the inclusion of a barometric pressure sensor proves beneficial as it measures the pressure exerted on the user's

S. Biswas, *Machine Learning and Deep Learning in Human Activity Recognition and Fall Detection*, Signals and Communication Technology,
https://doi.org/10.1007/978-3-032-09241-0_3

feet during walking, providing valuable information about gait [2, 12, 13] and weight distribution. This integrated approach to monitoring offers a comprehensive understanding of the user's activities and well-being, making it a promising solution for health care, fitness tracking, and enhancing overall quality of life. Furthermore, the paper critically examines existing literature, highlighting a gap in combining body vital monitoring with human activity recognition [14]. Most prior studies focused on a limited set of activities and did not consider the transitions between them. The integration of sensors, such as accelerometers, gyroscopes, and magnetometers, for both activity monitoring and body vital parameter tracking, is found to be lacking in current research. In response, our project proposes a sensor fusion approach [9], incorporating data from smartphones, smartwatches, oximeters, and blood pressure machines. This comprehensive strategy evaluates health parameters, diverse daily activities [15], and employs advanced algorithms to predict the individual's fitness level, categorizing them for tailored healthcare management. This innovative combination of sensor fusion [8, 9] and diverse activity monitoring offers a promising avenue for improving elderly care, disease prediction [16], and overall well-being.

3.2 State-of-the-Art Literatures: A Comprehensive Study

The existing literatures are mostly either focused on body vital monitoring/health monitoring or focused on human activity recognition. But if we can combine a person's movement data with body vital parameters, then this combination of data can be applied toward disease predictions and identification along with the monitoring. In the existing papers, we have found that they focused only on monitoring few human activities like sit, stand, walk, upstairs, downstairs, running, etc. [17, 18]. Most of the existing papers have not taken into consideration about transitions while changing from one activity to another the person is performing. What significant information could be extracted from in-between transitions? If a person prefers to avoid sitting on floor from stand position or takes unusually longer time in transition from stand to sit on floor, then the person might have gait issue or waist joint pain issue [19]. The sensors used while monitoring the activities are mostly accelerometer, gyroscope, and magnetometer. The combination of sensors for activity monitoring along with finding the change in body vital parameters is also not found in most of the existing papers (Table 3.1).

3.2.1 Sensors Used

We used different wearable sensors for monitoring the postures along with the body vital parameters [20]. The sensors with the help of which we have monitored different body vital parameters along with postures as follows. For each record in the dataset, it is provided:

Table 3.1 Table to compare the work performed and the proposed work

Work considered	Contribution	Sensors used	Limitations	Activities considered	Body vital considered	Classifier	Accuracy
Toward physical activity recognition using smartphone sensors [4]	Evaluation of sensors for different body positions and activities	Smartphone accelerometer, gyroscope, and magneto meter	The paper acknowledges that the dataset used for the experiments is limited to four participants and only includes six physical activities	Walking, running, sitting, standing, walking upstairs, and walking downstairs	Body vital is not considered	Naïve Bayes (NB), decision tables (DT), support vector machines (LSM)	It states that the overall results were fair
Human activities recognition in Android smartphone using support vector machine [7]	This offers the potential for applications in various fields, particularly in monitoring and health care	Accelerometer, gyroscope, accelerometer sensor linearity	In order to improve the system's performance and increase its detection capabilities, further research is required	Walking, standing, sitting, lying down, going up the stairs, and going down the stairs	The document does not provide specific details about the body vital signs being considered	Support vector machines (SVMs)	The system achieved an average accuracy of 89%

(continued)

Table 3.1 (continued)

Work considered	Contribution	Sensors used	Limitations	Activities considered	Body vital considered	Classifier	Accuracy
Development of a wearable sensor system for quantitative gait analysis [2]	The aim of the paper is to propose a motion analysis system with intelligent calibration for quantitative gait analysis, including gait phase detection	Gyroscope s (ENC05EB) and two-axis ADXL202 accelerometer are incorporated in this wearable sensor system	The gyroscopes used in the sensor system are prone to drift errors when worn on the human body. This can lead to cumulative errors in the analysis of multistep walking motions	Various physical activities related to walking. including initial contact, loading response, mid stance, terminal stance, pre swing, initial swing, mid swing, and terminal swing	It focuses on using gyroscopes and accelerometers to measure the angular velocity and inclination of leg segments during gait analysis	The wearable sensor system for quantitative gait analysis uses intelligent calibration and inference techniques for classification	The system has been validated through experiments and has shown high consistency and accuracy when compared to optical motion analysis systems
Identifying typical physical activity on smartphone with varying positions and orientations [15]	The paper discusses the feasibility and effectiveness of wearable sensors in activity classification	Accelerometer, gyroscope, and magnetic	The limitations of the paper include the fact that important activities such as going upstairs and downstairs were not studied	Standing, walking, upstairs, downstairs, and running	The study did not consider body vitals	Decision trees (J48), Naïve Bayes, and sequential minimal optimization (SMO)	Overall accuracy of 89.6% for the five activities

(continued)

Table 3.1 (continued)

Work considered	Contribution	Sensors used	Limitations	Activities considered	Body vital considered	Classifier	Accuracy
User, device, and orientation independent human activity recognition on mobile phones [17]	Multiple sensors are used to improve recognition accuracy	Accelerometer, gyroscope, and magnetic field sensors	The orientation of the smartphone affects the accuracy of activity recognition	Running, standing, biking, sitting, and walking	No, the document did not consider the recognition of body vital signs or measurements	K-nearest neighbors (KNN)	The accuracy of the proposed methodology for activity recognition using smartphone was 97%
Activity recognition with smartphone support [14]	It demonstrates the feasibility of accurately inferring human activity using just five features from two accelerometers	A triaxial accelerometer integrated into a Samsung Galaxy S GT-I9000 smartphone and a PLUX chest sensor	The placement of the smartphone in the participant's pocket and the chest sensor on the chest strap may vary, leading to variations in the recorded data	Sitting, standing, lying, walking, running, and cycling	The body vitals that were considered in the study were the triaxial accelerometer readings from the thigh and sternum	Decision tree, CART, SVM, multilayer perceptions, and Naïve Bayes	The custom classifier achieved an overall classification rate of 89%
Proposed work	The combination of sensors for activity monitoring along with finding the change in body vital parameters	A triaxial accelerometer, gyroscope, temperature sensor, pressure sensor, optoelectronic sensor	Disease prediction is not done, and more data needs to be collected	Sitting on chair, standing, sitting on floor, walking, upstairs, and downstairs	Body vitals are considered	Random forest, decision tree, and KNN	It is showing a very good accuracy

1. Triaxial acceleration from the accelerometer (*Ax*, *Ay*, *Az*)
2. Triaxial angular velocity from the gyroscope (*Gx*, *Gy*, *Gz*)
3. Body temperature (temperature sensors like thermocouples, thermistor, and resistance temperature detector present in digital thermometer)
4. Oxygen saturation of blood, i.e., SpO_2 (optoelectronic sensor present in oximeter)
5. Pulse rate (optoelectronic sensor present in oximeter)
6. Systolic blood pressure (pressure sensor present in digital blood pressure machine)
7. Diastolic blood pressure (pressure sensor present in digital blood pressure machine).

We first monitored the different health parameters like blood pressure, pulse rate, oxygen level in blood, body temperature, etc., of individual person in static position, i.e., sitting on chair. After performing the dynamic activities in 100 s of sliding window, we again measure their all health parameters. While monitoring the activities, we found that the young people performed all the activities within the time range but the time taken for elderly people to perform the activities is more as compared to young people [21, 22]. We found that they are unable to perform or reluctant to perform some activities like jogging, sitting on floor, etc. Hence, the difference occurs in the number of transitions between the old and young people within same time window while performing the activities. Also, immediately after performing the activities, there is a change in the body vital parameters considered such as blood pressure and pulse rate. Based on the number of activities performed and the values of the health parameter, our target is to predict whether the person is fit or not. If the person is unfit, then he/she needs to consult to doctor might be he/she is suffering from any health issue like heart problem or gait problem, etc. (Figs. 3.1, 3.2, 3.3 and 3.4).

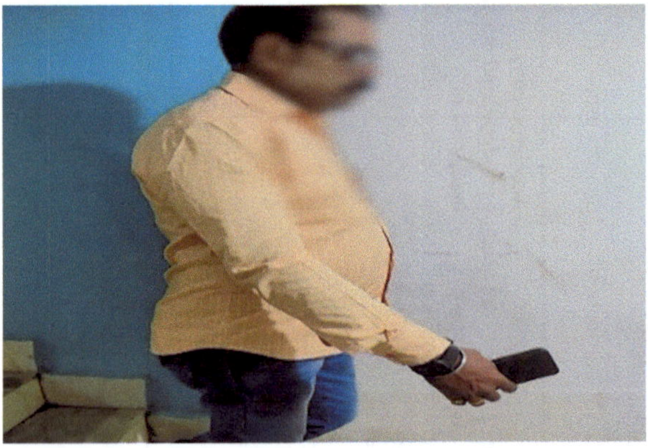

Fig. 3.1 Person performing the dynamic activities

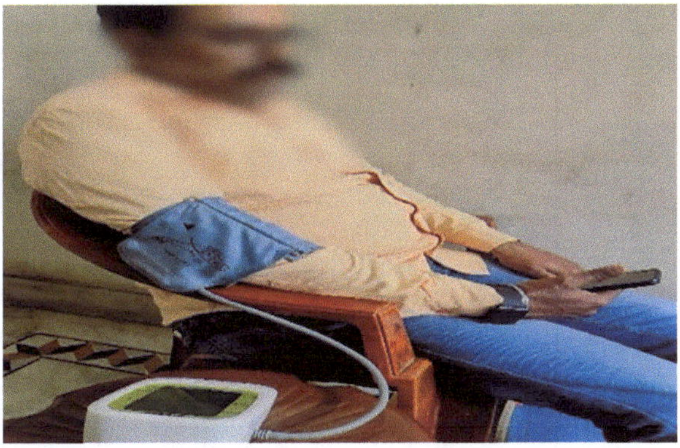

Fig. 3.2 Measuring the health parameters after performing the activities

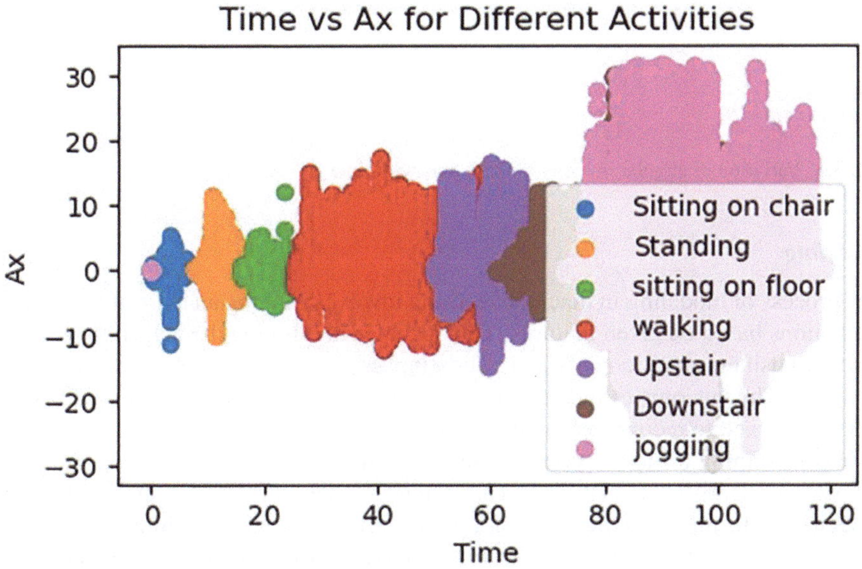

Fig. 3.3 Variation of acceleration along x-axis with time

3.2.2 Data Preprocessing

Data preprocessing is a crucial step in machine learning, encompassing tasks such as cleaning, transforming, and organizing raw data into a format suitable for model training [23, 24]. The specific preprocessing steps are contingent on the unique characteristics of the dataset and the requirements of the machine learning models being employed. Common practices include addressing missing values through removal or imputation using methods like mean, median, or advanced imputation techniques.

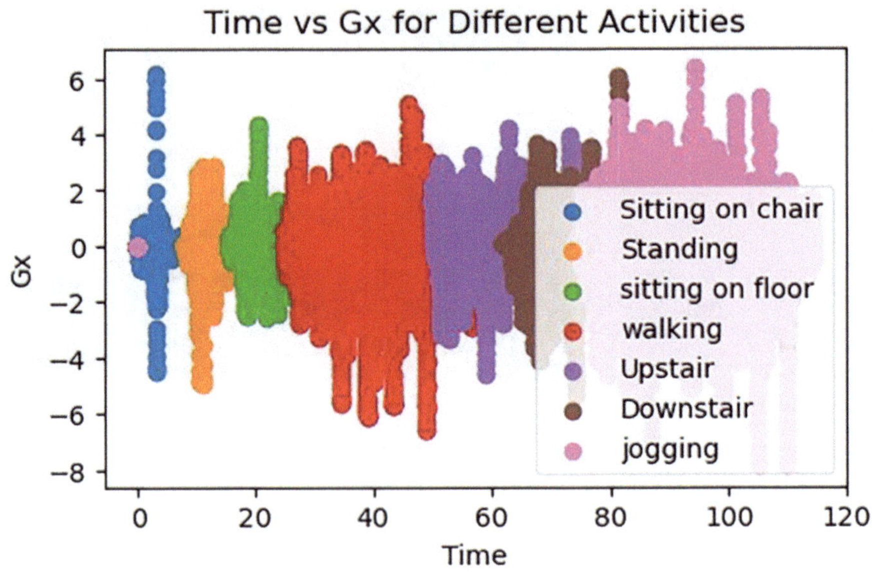

Fig. 3.4 Variation of angular velocity along x-axis with time

Modeling

The process of modeling in machine learning involves training an algorithm to make predictions based on given features. This includes fine-tuning the algorithm to meet specific business requirements and validating its performance on a separate set of data [25]. The outcome of the modeling process is a trained model, essentially a file that has learned to recognize specific patterns within the provided data.

When training a model, you expose it to a dataset and give it an algorithm to analyze and learn from that data. The trained model can then be applied to new, unseen data to make predictions. In simpler terms, it is like teaching a computer to recognize certain patterns so that it can make informed predictions when faced with new information [25]. This way, the model becomes a valuable tool for making predictions and reasoning over data in various applications (Fig. 3.5).

Fig. 3.5 Training and evaluating the model

3.2.3 Classification

Several efficient machine learning models [26, 27] are there to perform classification of activities irrespective of it is static or dynamic, simple or complex, single or concurrent, single user or multiusers associated with the activity, indoor, or outdoor, etc. Few of the ML models are described below:

Support Vector Machine (SVM)

A support vector machine (SVM) is a straightforward supervised machine learning algorithm mainly applied for classification tasks and occasionally for regression. The outcomes of each classifier will indicate whether the data point belongs to that specific class or not. This approach allows SVM to handle and effectively address problems involving more than two classes.

Decision Tree

A decision tree stands out as a robust [28] and widely used tool for classification and prediction tasks. It takes the form of a tree-like structure, resembling a flowchart. In this structure, each internal node signifies a test conducted on a specific attribute, each branch represents the potential outcome of that test, and each leaf node, also known as a terminal node, holds a class label. The process of creating a decision tree involves splitting the original dataset into subsets based on tests conducted on attribute values.

Random Forest

Random forest is a supervised learning algorithm that constructs an ensemble of decision trees using a technique called "bagging." The term "forest" refers to this collection of decision trees, and the bagging method [29] involves training these trees in combination. By aggregating the predictions of multiple trees, random forest provides a more robust and reliable solution.

k-Nearest Neighbors

The k-nearest neighbors algorithm, often referred to as KNN, is a type of supervised learning classifier [30]. Its fundamental idea is based on the assumption that similar points tend to be close to each other in the feature space. In other words, if data points share similarities, they are likely to belong to the same group or category.

This paper presents human activity recognition based on fusion of different sensors. In this paper, we have tried to monitor different activities like sitting on the chair, standing or sitting on floor, walking, upstairs, downstairs, and jogging within 100 secs time window. The sensors present in smart phone that are accelerometers and gyroscope help to measure triaxial acceleration, trivial angular velocity. After performing all the activities, we measure different health parameters like blood pressure, pulse rate, and SpO_2 level based on the sensors present in smart watch or other devices.

Devices Used

- **Smartphone**
- **Smartwatch**
- **Oximeter**
- **Blood pressure machine**.

Based on the data collected by sensors present in the devices, we have prepared the dataset. We have also measured the number of transitions performed by individual person, and we have classified each health parameters into different classes (Fig. 3.6).

Depending on this classification values of systolic_BP, diastolic_BP, pulse, SpO_2, and the number of transition performed by individual persons, we have prepared the model using different machine learning algorithms, and our aim is to predict whether the person is "very fit", "moderately fit", "mildly unfit", and "unfit". We have found that some people did not able to perform some of the activities like jogging, sitting on floor, etc. Based on this, we can say that if the person is not able to perform few activities means he/she has some joint pain or waist pain, and hence he/she did not perform that activities. We are monitoring this vital body parameters along with the seven activities performed by the person, and based on that, we are predicting whether he/she is fit or unfit. If the person is found to be unfit, we can say that he/she needs to consult to doctor may be he/she is suffering from gait issue, heart problem, etc.

```
def classify_diastolic_bp(diastolic_bp):
    if diastolic_bp < 80:
        return 0  # Normal
    elif 80 <= diastolic_bp <= 89:
        return 2  # Elevated
    elif 90<=diastolic_bp<120:
        return 3  # Hypertension Stage 2
    else:
        return 4  # Hypertensive Crisis
```

```
def classify_systolic_bp(systolic_bp):
    if systolic_bp < 120:
        return 0  # Normal
    elif 120 <= systolic_bp <= 129:
        return 1  # Elevated
    elif 130 <= systolic_bp <= 139:
        return 2  # Hypertension Stage 1
    elif 140<=systolic_bp< 180:
        return 3  # Hypertension Stage 2
    else:
        return 4  # Hypertensive Crisis
```

```
def classify_spo2(spo2):
    if spo2 >= 95:
        return 0 #"Normal"
    elif 91 <= spo2 <= 94:
        return 1 #"Mild Hypoxemia"
    elif 86 <= spo2 <= 90:
        return 2 #"Moderate Hypoxemia"
    else:
        return 3 #"Severe Hypoxemia"
```

```
def classify_pulse_rate(pulse_rate):
    if pulse_rate >= 60 and pulse_rate < 100:
        return 0  # Normal Resting Pulse Rate
    elif pulse_rate < 60:
        return 1  # Bradycardia
    else:
        return 2  # Tachycardia
```

Fig. 3.6 Classification of different health parameters in different range, i.e., normal, mild, moderate, and severe

3.2.4 *Design of an Activity Monitoring System*

Sensor Fusion: Integrating accelerometers and gyroscopes sensor present in smartphone, sensor present in smartwatch, oximeter, and blood pressure machine sensors for a comprehensive data fusion (Fig. 3.7).

Health Parameters: Assessing various health parameters like blood oxygen levels (SpO_2), systolic and diastolic blood pressure, and pulse rate to create a detailed health profile.

Activities Considered: Analyzing a range of activities such as sitting on chair, standing, sitting on the floor, climbing upstairs, descending downstairs, and jogging for a nuanced understanding of daily physical routines.

Fitness Check: Utilizing advanced algorithms to predict an individual's fitness level, categorizing them as fit, moderately fit, mildly unfit, or unfit based on observed data.

By combining data from multiple sources and activities, our project offers a comprehensive yet easy-to-understand analysis of an individual's health and fitness. The integration of sensor information and diverse activities enables a personalized

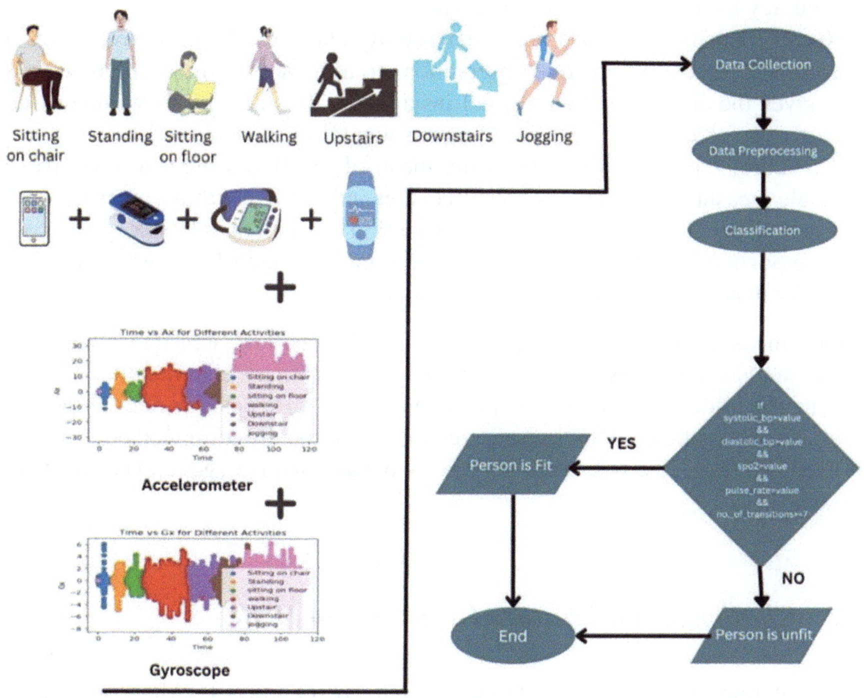

Fig. 3.7 Diagram to show all the activities and sensors used with the flowchart

assessment, providing users with actionable insights for making informed decisions about their well-being.

3.3 Performance Metrics

Measuring a HAR model's performance depends on the right metrics beyond the basic accuracy, particularly for unbalanced datasets or when errors of different types have different implications. The most standard metrics based on the confusion matrix [31–34] (true positives, true negatives, false positives, and false negatives) are as follows:

i. Accuracy: The ratio of the number of instances predicted correctly (both activities and non-activities) to the total number of instances. Although intuitive, accuracy is deceptive in imbalanced datasets, where the majority class overwhelms the predictions.
ii. Precision: Precision for a particular activity class is the ratio of correct positive predictions to total predicted positive observations. Precision replies to the question: "How many of all cases forecasted as this activity was correct?" High accuracy means low false positive rate.
iii. Recall (Sensitivity): For a particular activity class, recall is the proportion of correctly forecasted positive observations to all observations in the real class. It gives the answer to: "Of all real instances of this activity, how many were correctly forecasted?" High recall means low false negative rate.
iv. $F1$-Score: $F1$-score is the harmonic mean of recall and precision. It gives a single measure that averages both precision and recall and thus comes in handy when there is an imbalanced class distribution or when both false negatives and false positives need to be given equal importance. A high $F1$-score shows good performance with both precision and recall.

Other measurements such as specificity, ROC plots, and area under the curve (AUC) are also frequently employed, particularly in binary classification cases or assessing the trade-off between true positive rate and false positive rate. In the case of multiclass classification, these measurements are typically computed per class and then averaged (e.g., macro-average and micro-average) to give a general performance estimate.

3.3.1 Challenges and Future Directions in HAR

In spite of impressive progress, human activity recognition (HAR) continues to encounter a number of challenging problems that make large-scale deployment and best-possible performance in real-world, unconstrained settings difficult [35]. The resolution of these challenges is key to further development and real-world usefulness of HAR systems. At the same time, novel directions of research never cease to appear, which have the potential to extend HAR limits.

3.3.2 Data Collection and Annotation Challenges

One of the greatest challenges for HAR research is the tedious and frequently costly process of acquiring and precisely annotating large-scale, heterogeneous datasets. High-quality datasets are the lifeblood of machine learning, particularly for deep learning models that need enormous datasets to learn intricate patterns. But acquiring sensor data for HAR poses challenging problems:

i. Variability of Human Behavior: Human activities are naturally varied and done with considerable inter-subject (individual to individual) and intra-subject (same individual over time) variability. Individual activities can be influenced by age, gender, physical fitness, and even mood, making it difficult to capture all possible variations in a dataset.
ii. Contextual Dependence: One and the same physical movement could refer to varying activities based on context. Walking in the park is different from walking on a treadmill. It is difficult but essential to capture and integrate contextual information (location, time of day, presence of other people, etc.) for precise recognition.
iii. Annotation Burden: Annotating activities in streams of continuous sensor data manually is very time-consuming, labor-intensive, and susceptible to human error. It usually involves video recordings or direct observation, which creates privacy issues. The vagueness of activity boundaries (e.g., at what point does "sitting" stop and "standing" start?) makes annotation even more difficult.
iv. Imbalanced Datasets: Real-world activity datasets tend to be class-imbalanced, with frequent activities (e.g., sitting and standing) dominating the dataset over less frequent but potentially more important activities (e.g., falls and seizures). This imbalance can produce models that are good at predicting common activities but bad at predicting rare ones.
v. Privacy Concerns: Collecting sensitive data about individuals' movements and behaviors raises significant privacy and ethical concerns. Ensuring data anonymization, secure storage, and transparent usage policies are paramount.

Future directions in this area include developing more efficient and less intrusive data collection methodologies, leveraging semi-supervised or unsupervised learning techniques to reduce annotation reliance, and exploring synthetic data generation to augment real datasets.

3.3.3 Sensor Heterogeneity and Fusion

The vision of "all sensors" in HAR also comes with the inherent problem of sensor heterogeneity [35]. Most contemporary HAR systems aggregate information from hundreds of heterogeneous sensors, each having its own sampling rate, data type, noise signature, and units of measurement. Properly fusing all these heterogeneous data streams is a hard task.

i. Data Synchronization: Sensors tend to work in an asynchronous fashion, and synchronizing points of data from various sources in terms of time proves to be difficult. Meaningful data fusion requires precise synchronization.
ii. Feature-Level Fusion: Another typical method is to extract features separately from each sensor modality and concatenate the extracted features into one complete feature vector. Although simple, this approach may not capture very well the complex relationships and dependencies among various sensor modalities.
iii. Decision-Level Fusion: Here, every sensor modality is employed to train an individual activity recognition model, and the resultant activity prediction is obtained by fusing the individual models' output (decisions). This can include voting methods, weighted averaging, or more advanced ensemble learning methods. It will be resilient to a failure of a single sensor, but may fail to realize the full benefit of complementary information at an earlier point in processing.
iv. Deep Learning for Fusion: Deep learning frameworks, especially multimodal deep learning, hold great promise for sensor fusion. These can learn to extract and fuse features from diverse sensor data at different abstraction levels and may be able to identify intricate, nonlinear relationships that standard fusion techniques may not detect. Yet, developing and training them may be computationally demanding and need large and diverse sets of training data.

Future research will increasingly be driven toward more complex and adaptive sensor fusion methods, particularly those that use deep learning, to universally blend data from a constantly expanding set of sensing devices and environments.

3.4 Real-Time Processing and Computational Constraints

Most HAR applications, including fall detection, monitoring of the elderly, or interactive applications, need to provide real-time activity recognition. This puts strong computational demands on the HAR system, especially considering high-frequency sensor data and sophisticated machine learning models.

i. Latency Specifications: For serious use cases such as fall detection, the system has to detect an event and send an alert within a few milliseconds or seconds. This requires highly optimized hardware and algorithms.

ii. Resource-Constrained Devices: HAR is usually required to run on resource-constrained devices such as smartwatches, smartphones, or embedded systems that have slow processing power, limited memory, and low battery life. Deep learning models with high computational needs may not be easy to run on these devices.
iii. Edge Computing: In order to mitigate latency and privacy issues, there is an emerging trend of carrying out HAR computations near the source of the data, i.e., at the "edge" of the network, instead of exclusively using cloud computing. This requires the creation of light and efficient HAR models that can be executed well on edge devices.
iv. Model Optimization: Methods like model quantization, pruning, and knowledge distillation are being investigated to minimize the computational presence of deep learning models without drastically affecting accuracy. This enables their deployment in low-resource devices.

Energy-conscious and computationally light HAR algorithms and architectures will remain the focus of future work, as well as hardware acceleration and dedicated processing cores to facilitate ubiquitous real-time activity detection.

3.4.1 Privacy and Ethical Considerations

As HAR systems become more advanced and ubiquitous, with the growing utilization of vision-based and environmental sensors, strong privacy and ethical issues are presented. The day-to-day monitoring of people's actions creates a large volume of sensitive personal information, which, if misused, can cause privacy violations, information abuse, and discrimination.

i. Data Security and Anonymization: Secure storage and transmission of sensitive activity data is the top priority. Proper anonymization methods must be used to hide individual identities while enabling proper data analysis. It might prove difficult, though, to fully anonymize highly granular or multimodal data.
ii. Informed Consent: Ensuring that patients being monitored give truly informed consent is very important. Users must know what information is being captured, how it is going to be used, who will see it, and how long it will be kept. This is especially challenging in ambient sensing applications where the individuals may not be explicitly interacting with a device.
iii. Bias and Fairness: HAR models, as with any machine learning solution, can inherit and exacerbate bias in the training data. Where datasets are representative of heterogeneous populations, models may perform badly for specific demographic groups, resulting in unfair or erroneous activity recognition. Maintaining fairness and reducing bias in HAR systems is a significant ethical concern.
iv. Transparency and Explainability: The "black box" character of numerous deep learning models can complicate the identification of the reasons behind a specific

activity's recognition. In critical applications (e.g., health care), explainable AI (XAI) methods must be applied to ensure transparency and trust in HAR systems.

v. Abuse of Data: Misuse of HAR data for surveillance, targeted advertising, or even discrimination at the insurance or employment level is a serious issue. Strong regulatory measures and ethical standards are in place to avoid misuse.

Upcoming HAR research needs to incorporate privacy-friendly machine learning methods more and more, create sound ethical standards, and emphasize user-centered design so that these strong tools are responsibly developed and applied.

3.4.2 Emerging Trends and Open Research Questions

The domain of human activity recognition is dynamically changing due to innovations in sensor technology, machine learning methods, and computing capacities. Some of the emerging trends and open issues are defining the future of HAR [36, 37]:

i. Personalized HAR Models: Appreciating the large inter-subject variability, researchers are increasingly interested in creating personalized HAR models that learn to adapt to different users. This includes methods such as transfer learning, few-shot learning, and meta-learning to fine-tune universal models using small user-specific data.
ii. Unsupervised and Self-supervised Learning: Due to the difficulties of annotating data, unsupervised and self-supervised learning methods are increasingly being considered. These methods seek to learn semantically relevant representations from unlabeled sensor data, minimizing the dependency on expensive manual annotation.
iii. Ongoing Learning and Adaptation: Real-world settings are dynamic, and human activities may evolve over time. Ongoing learning (or lifelong learning) seeks to build HAR models that learn and adapt continuously to new activities, users, or settings without forgetting prior knowledge.
iv. Explainable AI (XAI) for HAR: As HAR models become more complex, understanding their decision-making process is crucial for trust and debugging. XAI techniques are being developed to provide insights into which sensor features or temporal patterns contribute most to an activity prediction.
v. Contextual Information Integration: In addition to raw sensor data, the incorporation of rich contextual information (e.g., calendar events, social interactions, and environmental conditions) has the potential to greatly improve HAR accuracy and enable a better insight into human behavior. There is ongoing research into integrating and harnessing such varied data sources effectively.
vi. Privacy-Preserving HAR: With growing privacy issues, efforts are under way to create HAR systems that can identify activities without compromising user privacy. These involve methods such as federated learning, differential privacy, and homomorphic encryption.

vii. Edge AI and On-Device Learning: The need for low-latency, real-time HAR is propelling research into deploying and training HAR models directly on edge devices (e.g., wearables and smartphones). This minimizes dependence on cloud infrastructure and improves privacy.
viii. Activity Forecasting and Anomaly Detection: Beyond simple recognition, future HAR systems will forecast future activities or identify unusual behaviors that are outside normal patterns, with important ramifications for anticipatory health care and security.
ix. Multimodal and Cross-Modal HAR: Continued investigation of the integration of data from very heterogeneous sensors (e.g., integrating physiological, inertial, and environmental data) and even cross-modal learning (e.g., training on vision data and transferring to sensor data) will remain a top research priority.

Solving these open problems and capitalizing on new trends will lead to more rational, responsive, and user-focused human activity recognition systems that can effortlessly intertwine into and augment our everyday lives.

3.5 Conclusion

The future scope of this research encompasses the development of real-time monitoring systems for continuous tracking of activities and vital parameters. Further exploration into additional sensors aims to enhance the accuracy and broaden the scope of health monitoring. Additionally, the investigation of personalized intervention strategies, tailored to individual fitness levels based on identified health parameters, holds promise for advancing the field. **Continuous Monitoring**: Develop real-time monitoring systems for ongoing tracking of activities and vital parameters. **Sensor Integration**: Explore additional sensors to enhance monitoring accuracy and expand the scope of health assessment. **Transition Time, Count, Pattern over a Time Window**: Transition data in-between activities carries vital information regarding a person's health condition. If transition time elapsed in between two consecutive transitions is abnormally high, then the person may experience discomfort during transition. So transition time taken by the person while changing the postures may indicate if he/she is suffering from any gait issue, etc. Also tendency to skip any specific activity, e.g., sitting on floor, jogging, stairs up, or stairs down multiple times during data collection or breathing discomfort during dynamic activities may indicate the person's proneness toward arthritis, gait, or heart-related problems. So along with activities, detailed data analysis of in-between transitions is also significant in disease prediction and monitoring. The vital body parameters are monitored along with the seven activities performed by the person as mentioned above, and based on that, it can be predicted whether he/she is fit or unfit. If the person is found to be unfit, we can say that he/she need to consult to doctor may be he/she is suffering from gait issue, heart problem, etc.

References

1. Kumar, P., Chauhan, S., & Awasthi, L. K. (2024). Human activity recognition (HAR) using deep learning: Review, methodologies, progress and future research directions. *Archives of Computational Methods in Engineering, 31*(1), 179–219.
2. Fu, B., et al. (2020). Sensing technology for human activity recognition: A comprehensive survey. *IEEE Access, 8*, 83791–83820.
3. Contoli, C., Freschi, V., & Lattanzi, E. (2024). Energy-aware human activity recognition for wearable devices: A comprehensive review. *Pervasive and Mobile Computing, 104*, 101976.
4. Thakur, D., & Biswas, S. (2020). Smartphone based human activity monitoring and recognition using ML and DL: A comprehensive survey. *Journal of Ambient Intelligence and Humanized Computing, 11*(11), 5433–5444.
5. Lara, O. D., & Labrador, M. A. (2012). A survey on human activity recognition using wearable sensors. *IEEE Communications Surveys & Tutorials, 15*(3), 1192–1209.
6. De-La-Hoz-Franco, E., et al. (2018). Sensor-based datasets for human activity recognition—A systematic review of literature. *IEEE Access, 6*, 59192–59210.
7. Mittal, P. (2022). Machine learning (ML) based human activity recognition model using smart sensors in IoT environment. In *2022 12th International Conference on Cloud Computing, Data Science & Engineering (Confluence)*. IEEE.
8. Mehmood, K., Imran, H. A., & Latif, U. (2020). HARDenseNet: A 1D DenseNet inspired convolutional neural network for human activity recognition with inertial sensors. In *2020 IEEE 23rd International Multitopic Conference (INMIC)*. IEEE.
9. Mishra, R., et al. (2024). Optimizing activity recognition through dominant axis identification in inertial sensors. IEEE Sensors Letters.
10. Rezaei, A., et al. (2022). An unobtrusive human activity recognition system using low resolution thermal sensors, machine and deep learning. *IEEE Transactions on Biomedical Engineering, 70*(1), 115–124.
11. FFT spectrum spread with machine learning (ML) analysis of triaxial acceleration from shirt pocket and torso for sensing coughs while walking.
12. Wang, Z., et al. (2023). Recognition of approximate motions of human based on micro-Doppler features. *IEEE Sensors Journal, 23*(11), 12388–12397.
13. Sassi, M., et al. (2024). Classification of shoulder rehabilitation exercises by using wearable systems and machine learning algorithms. *IEEE Sensors Journal, 24*(14), 22934–22944.
14. Tabrizi, S. S., Pashazadeh, S., & Javani, V. (2020). Comparative study of table tennis forehand strokes classification using deep learning and SVM. *IEEE Sensors Journal, 20*(22), 13552–13561.
15. Ehrnsperger, M. G., et al. (2020). Real-time gesture detection based on machine learning classification of continuous wave radar signals. *IEEE Sensors Journal, 21*(6), 8310–8322.
16. Nalwaya, A., Das, K., & Pachori, R. B. (2024) An automated framework for human emotion detection from multichannel EEG signals. *IEEE Sensors Journal, 24*(13), 20920–20927.
17. Thakur, D., & Biswas, S. (2021). Feature fusion using deep learning for smartphone based human activity recognition. *International Journal of Information Technology, 13*(4), 1615–1624.
18. Ankalaki, S. (2024). Simple to complex, single to concurrent sensor-based human activity recognition: Perception and open challenges. *IEEE Access, 12*, 93450–93486.
19. Zhang, L., et al. (2024). A multi-channel hybrid deep learning framework for multi-sensor fusion enabled human activity recognition. *Alexandria Engineering Journal, 91*, 472–485.
20. Athota, R. K., & Sumathi, D. (2022). Human activity recognition based on hybrid learning algorithm for wearable sensor data. *Measurement: Sensors, 24*, 100512.
21. Ghate, V., & Hemalatha, C. S. (2023). A comprehensive comparison of machine learning approaches with hyper-parameter tuning for smartphone sensor-based human activity recognition. *Measurement: Sensors, 30*, 100925.

22. Garcia-Gonzalez, D., et al. (2023). New machine learning approaches for real-life human activity recognition using smartphone sensor-based data. *Knowledge-Based Systems, 262*, 110260.
23. Imanzadeh, S., Tanha, J., & Jalili, M. (2024). Ensemble of deep learning techniques to human activity recognition using smart phone signals. *Multimedia Tools and Applications, 83*(42), 89635–89664.
24. Choudhury, N. A., & Soni, B. (2024). In-depth analysis of design & development for sensor-based human activity recognition system. *Multimedia Tools and Applications, 83*(29), 73233–73272.
25. Mallik, M., Sarkar, G., & Chowdhury, C. (2024). A deep learning framework for smartphone based human activity recognition. *Mobile Networks and Applications, 29*(1), 29–41.
26. Duan, H., et al. (2024). Wearable-based behaviour interpolation for semi-supervised human activity recognition. *Information Sciences, 665*, 120393.
27. Mani, N., Haridoss, P., & George, B. (2023). Evaluation of a combined conductive fabric-based suspender system and machine learning approach for human activity recognition. *IEEE Open Journal of Instrumentation and Measurement, 2*, 1–10.
28. Raziani, S., & Azimbagirad, M. (2022). Deep CNN hyperparameter optimization algorithms for sensor-based human activity recognition. *Neuroscience Informatics, 2*(3), 100078.
29. Gupta, S. (2021). Deep learning based human activity recognition (HAR) using wearable sensor data. *International Journal of Information Management Data Insights, 1*(2), 100046.
30. Saidani, O., et al. (2023). An efficient human activity recognition using hybrid features and transformer model. *IEEE Access, 11*, 101373–101386.
31. Vinod, P. R., & Anitha, A. (2023). A novel human activity recognition model for smartphone authentication. *Wireless Personal Communications, 129*(4), 2791–2812.
32. Ek, S., Portet, F., & Lalanda, P. (2023). Transformer-based models to deal with heterogeneous environments in human activity recognition. *Personal and Ubiquitous Computing, 27*(6), 2267–2280.
33. Waqar, S., & Pätzold, M. (2023). A simulation-based framework for the design of human activity recognition systems using radar sensors. *IEEE Internet of Things Journal, 11*(8), 14494–14507.
34. Mohsen, S. (2023). Recognition of human activity using GRU deep learning algorithm. *Multimedia Tools and Applications, 82*(30), 47733–47749.
35. Qiu, S., Zhao, H., Jiang, N., Wang, Z., Liu, L., An, Y., et al. (2022). Multi-sensor information fusion based on machine learning for real applications in human activity recognition: State-of-the-art and research challenges. *Information Fusion, 80*, 241–265.
36. Guo, W., Yamagishi, S., & Jing, L. (2024). Human activity recognition via Wi-Fi and inertial sensors with machine learning. *IEEE Access, 12*, 18821–18836.
37. Ihianle, I. K., et al. (2020). A deep learning approach for human activities recognition from multimodal sensing devices. *IEEE Access, 8*, 179028–179038.

Chapter 4
Deep Learning in HAR

4.1 Introduction

Human activity recognition (HAR)-based research has got immense popularity in the research community enabled with rapid growth in enabling technologies such as sensors, embedded systems, high speed Internet 5G, cloud computing, machine learning, deep learning, and neural networks. HAR is a specific field of research that emphasizes on finding movement patterns of human being by analyzing sensor-based motion data. Deep learning in HAR has made it more attractive to the research community because of its ability to develop intelligent frameworks for lifestyle monitoring, personalized health care, activities of daily living, disease detection [1, 2], etc.

Using wearable, ambient, or vision-based sensors, raw movement data is collected through accelerometers, gyroscope, and magnetometers embedded in wearable devices. The huge time-series data captured during movement of human being such as walk, stand, sit, jump, stairs up, and stairs down, and the data collection goes on using sensors embedded in smartphones, smart watches, or dedicated wearable devices. This activity identification and activity pattern recognition of specific users have immense applications in enhancing and ensuring quality living of people specifically diseased elderly [3, 4].

Machine learning-based HAR has a long time reference but deep learning-based HAR frameworks are nowadays more preferred because of its advantages over machine learning. Machine extracts features, e.g., mean, variance, entropy, FFT, and correlation of accelerometer/gyroscope signals through manual feature engineering methods which require domain-specific preprocessing. Performances of the ML-based HAR models in terms of accuracy, precision, recall, $F1$-score, confusion matrix, etc., majorly depend on the handcrafted features quality. In contrast, deep learning replaces the rigorous task of manual feature extraction with automatic hierarchical feature learning directly from raw sensor data. These characteristics are

S. Biswas, *Machine Learning and Deep Learning in Human Activity Recognition and Fall Detection*, Signals and Communication Technology,
https://doi.org/10.1007/978-3-032-09241-0_4

immensely useful in the context of a diversified activity and patient or human subject in concern [5] to ensure improved recognition accuracy.

When health monitoring, disease detection, disease prediction, rehabilitation monitoring of patients are under consideration, deep learning-based HAR models win over machine learning-based models. Recent state-of-the-art research shows that in health monitoring and care applications, use of CNN, LSTM, and hybrid frameworks to processes is increasing remarkably to process sequential sensory data to capture both spatial and temporal dependencies which are critical in health monitoring [6].

Different diseases can be detected with enhanced accuracy using deep learning-based HAR models, and few are mentioned below.

In diseases like neuro degenerative disorders such as Parkinson's disease (PD), deep learning has immense applications in reference to recent literatures. Here different disease symptoms such as tremors, gait freezing, and reduced movement speed could be identified with automated feature learning techniques. Patterns related to gait signals, step or walk patterns, hand tremors, etc., could be identified with very high accuracy and are helpful in Parkinson's disease (PD) detection. Another very much prevalent disease in this category is Alzheimer's or dementia, highly relevant in senior people over 60. Dominating symptoms of this disease are irregular movement patterns, disorientation, wandering in nature, etc., and HAR can detect abnormal activity routine that could be relatable with symptoms such as repeated walking loops and restlessness.

Musculoskeletal disorders like arthritis, osteoporosis, joint injuries, back pain, etc., affect movement, gait, posture, and mobility. HAR detects physical activities such as walking, sitting, and standing and identifies abnormal gait patterns, reduced range of motion, or irregular postures. Through continuous daily activities tracking, the deep learning models evaluate disease progression or recovery after surgery/ rehabilitation. Deep learning-based HAR frameworks are getting increasing popularity because of its noninvasive nature, beneficial in real-time monitoring outside clinical settings, and ensure early detection of abnormal movement before severe disability, personalized treatment in terms of rehabilitation, and appropriate feedback facility for clinicians and patients.

As per WHO report, due to majorly lifestyle disorders, environmental pollutions etc., cardiovascular and respiratory diseases [7] are alarmingly increasing and in post-COVID era, these diseases are very much prevalent in senior elderly. Symptoms such as lethargy in physical dynamic activities, short of breather, and fatigue could be detected combining motion sensor data and health vitals sensors data such as heart rate sensor, pulse rate sensor, and SpO_2 sensor, i.e., sensor fusion-based methods. Deep learning-based smart health frameworks are also being efficiently utilized in rehabilitation monitoring after chronic and critical diseases such as stroke, heart attack by analyzing changes in activity patterns in terms of smoothness, symmetry, activity levels, etc.

Moreover, the unobtrusive nature of sensor-based monitoring encourages consistent data collection, making it easier for clinicians to gain insights into patient health over time. This abstract highlights the transformative role of deep learning in advancing HAR applications for disease detection, suggesting a promising future for intelligent, data-driven healthcare solutions. In summary, the fusion of deep learning models with HAR techniques is transforming the landscape of disease detection and patient care. By enabling continuous, intelligent health monitoring, this interdisciplinary approach holds tremendous potential to enhance early diagnosis, personalize treatments, and ultimately improve health outcomes across a wide spectrum of diseases.

4.2 Types of Deep Learning Models Used in HAR

Deep learning models have become foundational in disease detection due to their ability to learn complex patterns from large, high-dimensional datasets such as sensor signals, medical images, and time-series health data. In the context of human activity recognition (HAR), these models process continuous streams of data from wearable sensors to detect abnormalities that may indicate the presence or progression of a disease. Below are the key types of deep learning models widely applied in this field.

4.2.1 Convolutional Neural Networks (CNNs)

CNNs are primarily used to extract spatial features from structured data and have been adapted successfully for time-series sensor data in HAR. They automatically learn filters to detect patterns such as irregular gait or tremors—common in neurological conditions like Parkinson's disease. In multichannel sensor systems, CNNs can efficiently analyze multiple data streams (e.g., from accelerometers and gyroscopes) to detect subtle movement disorders, for an example, early detection of Parkinson's disease by identifying tremor patterns or gait instability from wrist or foot sensors.

Reference [3] introduces a hybrid model combining CNNs and long short-term memory (LSTM) networks to process multimodal data from wearable sensors. The CNN layers extract spatial features from raw sensor inputs, while the LSTM layers capture temporal dependencies. Evaluated on the Opportunity dataset, the model achieved superior performance compared to traditional methods, highlighting the effectiveness of deep learning in HAR tasks. The authors propose an ensemble of deep LSTM networks for activity recognition using wearable sensor data. While primarily focusing on LSTM architectures, the study underscores the importance of deep learning models in capturing complex temporal patterns inherent in human activities, setting a foundation for integrating CNNs in such frameworks [8]. One more study applies CNNs directly to raw accelerometer data from mobile devices for activity recognition [9]. By transforming time-series data into a format suitable for CNN processing, the model eliminates the need for manual feature extraction. The approach demonstrates high accuracy on multiple datasets, showcasing CNNs' capability in handling sensor-based HAR. Another study presents a deep CNN model tailored for multichannel time-series data from wearable sensors [10].

By employing multiple convolutional layers, the model captures intricate patterns across different sensor channels. The approach achieves notable accuracy improvements over traditional methods, emphasizing CNNs' strength in processing complex sensor data. The research introduces a multimodal CNN architecture that integrates data from various sensors, such as accelerometers and gyroscopes, for activity recognition in Ref. [11]. By processing each modality through separate CNN branches before fusion, the model effectively captures complementary information, leading to enhanced recognition performance. In Ref. [12], a comprehensive survey reviews deep learning approaches, including CNNs, for sensor-based activity recognition. It discusses various architectures, training strategies, and applications in health care. The paper highlights the advantages of CNNs in automatic feature extraction and their adaptability to different sensor modalities. The authors propose a method combining 2D pose estimation with CNNs to recognize human activities from video data. By extracting skeletal keypoints and feeding them into a CNN, the model effectively identifies activities relevant to healthcare monitoring, such as fall detection, demonstrating the versatility of CNNs beyond traditional sensor data [4]. A study discussed in Ref. [13] presents a residual CNN architecture designed for HAR in smart healthcare environments. The residual connections facilitate deeper network training by mitigating vanishing gradient issues. Evaluated on multiple datasets, the model achieves high accuracy, confirming the benefits of residual learning in HAR tasks. Another group has introduced a hybrid model combining multiple CNN and RNN branches to process different sensor modalities. Each CNN head extracts features from a specific modality, which are then fused and passed through RNN layers for temporal modeling. This architecture effectively captures both spatial and temporal aspects of human activities [14]. A review paper discusses various deep learning algorithms [15, 16], including CNNs, for HAR using mobile and wearable sensors. It examines the strengths and limitations of different models, data preprocessing techniques, and deployment challenges in healthcare settings. The paper provides insights into future research directions for CNN-based HAR systems.

4.2.2 Recurrent Neural Networks (RNNs)

RNNs are designed to process sequential data, making them well-suited for analyzing time-series signals. Unlike CNNs, RNNs consider the temporal dynamics of activities—crucial in recognizing how movements evolve over time, for an example, monitoring physical activity changes in patients with Alzheimer's disease to detect early cognitive decline.

In [12], authors introduced SLOTH, an architecture designed for online gesture recognition using wearable triaxial accelerometers. The system employs a recurrent neural network (RNN) probabilistic classifier coupled with a continuous gesture detection mechanism. This approach ensures high precision and recall in real-time scenarios, making it suitable for applications requiring immediate system reactivity, such as assistive robotics and interactive healthcare systems. Reference [17] proposed a deep neural network architecture that combines convolutional neural networks (CNNs) with long short-term memory (LSTM) networks and integrates a self-attention mechanism. This model captures spatio-temporal features from wearable sensor data and emphasizes important time points, enhancing activity recognition performance. The approach demonstrated significant improvements over traditional models across six public datasets, highlighting its potential for long-term health-care monitoring. In the study [18], a hybrid model combining CNNs and bidirectional gated recurrent units (BiGRUs) was developed for feature extraction, followed by a regularized extreme learning machine (RELM) for classification. The system achieved an average accuracy of 98.3% in classifying 18 physical activities using data from smartphones and smartwatches, demonstrating its effectiveness in mobile health (mHealth) applications. The paper in Ref. [19] presents a novel HAR method that first establishes an information gain-based model to determine optimal sensor placement based on human skeletal structure. Subsequently, an attention-based RNN is employed for activity classification. This approach addresses challenges related to sensor deployment variability and the complexity of deep learning models, offering a more standardized and efficient solution for wearable HAR systems. The study [20] focused on recognizing eating activities using smartwatch accelerometer data. By employing an LSTM-ANN architecture, the model achieved a 90% success rate in identifying individual bites, distinguishing them from other activities like smoking or jogging. This work underscores the potential of RNNs in monitoring specific health-related behaviors. Reference [21] introduced a deep network architecture that integrates residual connections with bidirectional LSTM cells. The residual connections facilitate gradient flow, mitigating the vanishing gradient problem, while the bidirectional LSTM captures temporal dependencies in both forward and backward directions. The model demonstrated improved accuracy on the Opportunity and UCI datasets, highlighting its robustness in HAR tasks. Another study combined CNNs and LSTM networks to leverage their respective strengths in spatial and temporal feature extraction. The hybrid model effectively recognized various human activities, emphasizing its applicability in health monitoring systems where understanding complex activity patterns is crucial [22]. Where the authors of [23] proposed a CNN-LSTM model tailored for healthcare monitoring applications. By integrating CNNs for spatial feature extraction and LSTMs for temporal analysis, the model achieved high accuracy in activity recognition tasks. The study's focus on real-life healthcare settings, such as remote patient monitoring and elderly care, underscores its practical relevance. Some group of researchers in study [24] has developed a deep recurrent neural network (DRNN) optimized for high-throughput HAR using raw accelerometer data. The model achieved recognition rates of 95.42% for single activity trials and 83.43% for multiple sequential activities, outperforming traditional methods. Its compact architecture and real-time processing capabilities make it suitable for mobile health applications. One study has been conducted by the authors of Ref. [17] for a comparative study of different RNN architectures, including simple RNN, LSTM, and GRU, for HAR tasks. By analyzing the impact of various hyperparameters, such as hidden units and sequence length, the study provides insights into optimizing RNN models for wearable sensor data, aiding in the development of efficient healthcare monitoring systems.

4.2.3 Long Short-Term Memory (LSTM) Networks

LSTMs are a special type of RNN that addresses the vanishing gradient problem, enabling the model to remember long-term dependencies in data. This makes LSTMs particularly effective in recognizing extended patterns in sensor data that may indicate chronic conditions. For illustration tracking post-stroke rehabilitation progress through prolonged monitoring of walking and hand movement patterns.

In Ref. [20], proposed a 4-layer CNN-LSTM hybrid model for HAR using smartphone sensor data. The model combines convolutional layers for spatial feature extraction with LSTM layers for temporal sequence modeling. Evaluated on the UCI-HAR dataset, the model achieved an accuracy of 99.39%, outperforming other LSTM-based architectures. Bayesian optimization was employed for hyperparameter tuning, enhancing model performance. The study discussed in Ref. [23] introduced a deep network architecture integrating residual connections with bidirectional LSTM cells. The residual connections facilitate gradient flow, mitigating the vanishing gradient problem, while the bidirectional LSTM captures temporal dependencies in both forward and backward directions. The model demonstrated improved accuracy on the Opportunity and UCI datasets, highlighting its robustness in HAR tasks. The authors of the research [8] proposed a novel method combining multi-head CNNs with LSTM layers for HAR. The multi-head CNNs extract features from different sensor modalities, which are then fused and passed through LSTM layers for temporal modeling. This approach achieved state-of-the-art accuracy, demonstrating the effectiveness of combining spatial and temporal features for HAR. Reference [24] addressed challenges in real-life HAR datasets, such as class imbalance and data quality issues, by developing ensembles of deep LSTM networks. By combining multiple LSTM learners, the ensemble approach improved recognition performance on datasets like Opportunity, PAMAP2, and Skoda, showcasing its potential for real-world applications. Another study has el tailored for healthcare monitoring applications. By integrating CNNs for spatial feature extraction and LSTMs for temporal analysis, the model achieved high accuracy in activity recognition tasks. The study's focus on real-life healthcare settings, such as remote patient monitoring and elderly care, underscores its practical relevance. The authors presented a HAR approach combining CNNs and LSTMs. In this hybrid approach, LSTMs are utilized in focusing on disentangling timing and ordering information within these features. CNN is utilized for automated feature learning through extraction and analysis of spatially distributed feature information. Using OWN and UCF-50 datasets [17], a number of experiments have been conducted for performance evaluation of proposed model. Performance enhancement in terms of accuracy and reliability utilizing feature fusion approach has been achieved in this method.

4.2.4 Gated Recurrent Units (GRUs)

GRUs are a simplified version of LSTMs, offering comparable performance with reduced computational complexity. They are ideal for mobile or real-time applications in health monitoring where processing power is limited. Real-time fall detection in elderly individuals may signal complications from osteoporosis or neurological issues.

Reference [18] proposed an innovative HAR method that integrates edge computing with a GRU-based deep learning network. The model, termed OI-EleAttG-GRU, combines an O-Inception convolutional structure with an element-wise attention gate-enhanced GRU. This architecture effectively reduces time complexity and enhances feature extraction. By offloading computation to edge servers, the system optimizes energy consumption and processing time on wearable devices. The model achieved an average accuracy of 85.4% on challenging HAR datasets, outperforming traditional RNN methods. A computationally efficient framework combining a dual attention CNN with a bidirectional GRU for HAR. The dual attention mechanism focuses on both channel and spatial features, enhancing the extraction of salient information from video frames. The bidirectional GRU captures temporal dependencies in both forward and backward directions. This architecture demonstrated significant improvements in execution time and recognition accuracy compared to contemporary methods. Reference [19] presented ECG-NETS, a hybrid model integrating capsule networks with modified GRUs (MGRUs) and extreme learning machines (ELMs) for HAR. The capsule networks extract spatial features, while MGRUs capture temporal dynamics. ELMs are employed for efficient training. Validated on real-time IoT data and the WISDM dataset, the model achieved superior performance with reduced computational complexity, making it suitable for IoT-based healthcare applications. Reference [25] networks to classify psychological stress levels based on ECG signals. Heart rate variability (HRV) features are extracted and fed into a deep GRU network, capturing temporal patterns associated with stress. The model achieved an estimation accuracy of 78%, outperforming other mainstream methods. This approach demonstrates the potential of GRUs in mental health monitoring using wearable devices. Reference [26] proposed DanHAR, a dual attention network that combines channel and temporal attention mechanisms with GRUs for multimodal HAR. The model effectively captures spatial–temporal dependencies from accelerometer and gyroscope data. Experiments on four public HAR datasets demonstrated that DanHAR achieves state-of-the-art performance with minimal parameter overhead, highlighting its efficiency and accuracy. Reference [18] introduced a GRU-based model enhanced with channel attention (CA) and temporal attention (TA) mechanisms for sensor-based HAR. The model processes time-sliced sensor data, applying CA to emphasize important sensor channels and TA to focus on relevant time steps. Evaluations showed that the combined attention mechanisms significantly improved recognition accuracy while maintaining low computational costs, making it suitable for real-time healthcare applications. Reference [19] introduced SiTGRU, a simplified GRU model designed for abnormality detection in sequential data. By removing the reset gate and replacing the hyperbolic tangent activation with a sigmoid function, SiTGRU reduces complexity while maintaining performance. Applied to the CUHK Avenue and UCSD datasets, the model outperformed standard GRU and LSTM networks, demonstrating its effectiveness in detecting anomalies in healthcare monitoring systems. Reference [27] proposed a multimodal attention network that integrates GRUs with attention mechanisms for HAR using wearable sensor data. The model effectively captures temporal dependencies and emphasizes relevant features across different sensor modalities. Experiments demonstrated improved recognition accuracy, showcasing the model's potential in healthcare applications. Reference [26] developed deep learning framework employing GRU networks for HAR. The model processes sequential sensor data to capture temporal patterns associated with various activities. Evaluations on benchmark datasets indicated that the GRU-based framework achieved high accuracy, highlighting its applicability in healthcare monitoring.

4.2.5 Deep Belief Networks (DBNs)

DBNs are composed of stacked restricted Boltzmann machines (RBMs) and are used for unsupervised feature learning. While less common today due to the popularity of CNNs and LSTMs, they have been applied in disease classification using activity data classifying types of motor impairments by learning latent features from movement signals.

Reference [28] introduced the HF-SPHR model, integrating hybrid features with a DBN for recognizing physical healthcare patterns. Utilizing datasets like mHealth and HuGaDB, the model achieved accuracies of 93.33% and 92.50%, respectively. The study highlighted the DBN's capability in distinguishing subtle differences in activities such as walking, running, and jogging, emphasizing its potential in healthcare monitoring systems. Reference [29] has developed a DBN-based approach for detecting and classifying falls among the elderly. By analyzing sensor data from smartphones, the model effectively differentiated between various fall types and daily activities. The research underscored the DBN's proficiency in handling complex patterns, making it suitable for real-time fall detection in healthcare settings. Reference [30] has proposed the IHPTDL-HAR technique, combining DBNs with Harris Hawks optimization for hyperparameter tuning. The model focused on recognizing human actions in healthcare environments, aiding in patient management. Experimental results demonstrated the model's superiority over existing methods, showcasing its applicability in medical services. Reference [31] introduced an error-based fuzzy dragon DBN, integrating fuzzy logic with DBNs to enhance activity recognition. By extracting hierarchical skeleton features from video data, the model achieved high accuracy in recognizing complex human activities. This approach highlighted the DBN's adaptability in processing diverse data types for healthcare applications. In the study discussed in Ref. [30], researchers combined HAR with diabetic retinopathy analysis to facilitate early diagnosis of Type 2 Diabetes Mellitus. By employing DBNs alongside other deep learning models, the system analyzed smartphone sensor data to monitor physical activities, contributing to proactive healthcare management. Reference [32] has developed a DBN-based model for HAR using data from wearable sensors. The study emphasized the DBN's capability in capturing temporal dependencies and complex patterns in sensor data, leading to improved accuracy in activity recognition tasks relevant to healthcare monitoring. Reference [33] has proposed a DBN model integrated with feature selection techniques to enhance HAR performance. By selecting relevant features from sensor data, the model achieved higher accuracy and reduced computational complexity, making it suitable for real-time healthcare applications. The DBN-based framework tailored for HAR in smart home environments. The model effectively recognized daily activities by analyzing data from ambient sensors, highlighting the DBN's potential in supporting independent living for the elderly and individuals with disabilities. The researchers have explored the integration of data augmentation methods with DBNs to improve HAR accuracy. By generating synthetic data to address class imbalance, the model demonstrated enhanced performance in recognizing various activities, contributing to more robust healthcare monitoring systems.

4.2.6 Autoencoders

Autoencoders are useful for anomaly detection and unsupervised learning. They compress input data into a latent space and then reconstruct it; deviations in reconstruction can signal abnormal behavior. Detecting irregular walking patterns that may precede a cardiovascular event or diabetic neuropathy.

Reference [34] has introduced a continuous autoencoder (CAE) model designed to enhance feature extraction from wearable sensor data for HAR. By incorporating Gaussian noise into the activation function, the CAE effectively modeled continuous data. The study achieved a 99.3% accuracy rate on a dataset comprising 19 activities, demonstrating the model's robustness in healthcare monitoring scenarios. The study employed in Ref. [35] in stacked denoising autoencoders (SDAEs) to automatically extract features from wearable sensor data, focusing on recognizing transitional activities crucial in health care, such as fall detection. The model outperformed traditional machine learning methods, highlighting the effectiveness of SDAEs in capturing complex activity patterns. Reference [36] has proposed a multi-input multi-output autoencoder (MIMO-AE) model utilizing channel state information (CSI) data for HAR. Here, classification accuracy is improved through fine-tuning of the autoencoder. To handle multilabel HAR tasks, a deep auto-set model combining autoencoders with set prediction networks has been introduced. Overlapping activities are important to analyze and understand patient behavior, and this contribution addresses the challenges of overlapping activities. The authors in [37] focused on performance enhancement of HAR framework by integrating convolutional autoencoders with advanced preprocessing techniques, which includes normalization and data balancing issues. A hierarchical self-attention autoencoder model is presented here to detect and recognize both known and unknown set of activities. It addresses the open-set recognition problem in HAR. Also, in ever-evolving HAR systems and behavioral patterns in patients, adaptive HAR is feasible with the ability of recognizing unknown human activities. Deep stacked autoencoder (DSAE) models are proposed to identify ADL activities with higher accuracy.

4.3 Convolutional Neural Networks (CNNs) Used for HAR-Related Disease Detection

CNN is not only used for human activity recognition, but also widely and successfully has been applied in healthcare disease detection as well. Some of the disease detection using CNN model is described below.

4.3.1 Parkinson's Disease Detection Using DaTscan Images

The researchers developed an ensemble of CNN models to classify DaTscan images for Parkinson's disease detection. The ensemble approach improved classification accuracy, demonstrating the effectiveness of combining multiple CNN architectures for medical image analysis.

Mallik et al. [6] proposed an ensemble-based deep learning approach to detect Parkinson's disease using DaTscan images. The researchers developed a framework that combines multiple convolutional neural network (CNN) models to improve diagnostic accuracy and reliability.

The study used a dataset of DaTscan images, which are commonly employed to visualize dopamine transporter activity in the brain—a key indicator in diagnosing Parkinson's disease. Prior to training, the images underwent preprocessing steps such as resizing, intensity normalization, and noise reduction to standardize input data and enhance feature extraction.

The authors selected several CNN architectures, including VGG16, ResNet50, and DenseNet121, which were fine-tuned through transfer learning. Each model was individually trained on the preprocessed dataset, and their outputs were combined through a majority voting ensemble strategy to produce the final classification. This ensemble method was used to reduce individual model bias and increase overall robustness.

To evaluate model performance, the authors used various metrics including accuracy, sensitivity, specificity, $F1$-score, and area under the ROC curve (AUC). Their ensemble approach outperformed individual CNN models in most metrics, demonstrating its effectiveness in detecting Parkinson's disease from neuroimaging data [10].

4.4 Datasets for Human Activity Recognition Applied with Deep Learning Techniques

This section details out the popularly used **datasets for applying deep learning models** in **human activity recognition (HAR)** research. Also which deep learning models have been applied on which dataset is also specified. Each entry includes dataset details and respective deep learning approaches applied.

4.4.1 UCI HAR Dataset and Deep Learning Models

Dataset Description: In UCI HAR dataset, 30 subjects performed 6 activities while carrying a smartphone with embedded accelerometer and gyroscope.

Activity Classes: Walking, sitting, standing, lying, and walking upstairs/downstairs.

Deep Learning Models Applied

CNN: for spatial feature extraction from time-series segments.

LSTM/Bi-LSTM: for capturing temporal dependencies.

CNN-LSTM hybrids: for spatial–temporal feature learning.

WISDM Dataset and Applied Deep Learning Models

Description: Smartphone-based accelerometer data from users performing activities with the phone in their pocket.

Deep Learning Models Applied

CNN: for recognizing motion patterns.

LSTM: to model time-series nature.

Deep Belief Networks (DBN): unsupervised pretraining.

4.4.2 MobiAct Dataset and Deep Learning

Description of Dataset: This dataset is prepared for fall detection and ADL (Activities of Daily Living), uses smartphones' IMU sensors.

Deep Learning Models That Have Been Applied in Existing Literatures

CNNs and deep feedforward networks.

LSTM and CNN-LSTM hybrids.

Autoencoders for anomaly detection.

HAPT Dataset: Includes activity and transition in between two activities.

Details of Dataset: Extended version of UCI HAR with 12 activities (6 ADLs and 6 transitions).

Deep Learning Models Already Applied in Different Works

1D CNNs for time series.

RNNs for activity transition detection.

4.5 Automatic Feature Extraction in Human Activity Recognition Using Deep Learning

Human activity recognition (HAR) involves identifying physical activities of individuals based on data captured from various sensors, such as accelerometers, gyroscopes, and ambient sensors. Traditionally, HAR systems relied heavily on handcrafted features extracted using domain knowledge and statistical methods. However, this process is time-consuming, often nontransferable, and prone to human bias. Deep learning techniques have revolutionized HAR by **enabling** automatic feature extraction directly from raw sensor data, reducing the need for manual feature engineering, and improving classification accuracy across diverse activity types and users. Deep learning models automatically learn hierarchical and discriminative features from raw input data. In HAR, this is particularly advantageous, as raw sensor signals (such as time-series accelerometer or gyroscope data) can be directly input into the network, which extracts relevant features through its layers during training.

4.5.1 Convolutional Neural Networks (CNNs)

CNNs are effective in learning **local temporal dependencies** and spatial patterns in multivariate time-series data. They automatically extract features such as signal peaks, periodicity, and local trends that are characteristic of different human activities.

Example: A 1D CNN applied to accelerometer data can learn motion patterns distinguishing walking from running without explicit signal transformation.

4.5.2 Recurrent Neural Networks (RNNs) and LSTM

RNNs, especially **long short-term memory (LSTM)** networks, are suitable for modeling **temporal dependencies** in sequential sensor data. They automatically learn how past sensor values influence current activity, capturing long-range dependencies and dynamic transitions.

Example: An LSTM model can distinguish between sitting and transitioning to standing by identifying temporal patterns across time steps.

4.5.3 Autoencoders

Autoencoders are unsupervised models that learn compact representations (latent features) of input data. In HAR, stacked autoencoders can extract abstract features that enhance the performance of downstream classifiers.

Example: Autoencoders trained on raw IMU data learn latent features that reflect signal dynamics without activity labels.

4.5.4 Hybrid Models (e.g., CNN-LSTM)

Combining CNN and LSTM layers leverages **spatial–temporal feature learning**—CNNs extract local features, while LSTMs model sequential dependencies. This approach is highly effective for complex or overlapping activities.

Example: CNN layers detect motion signatures, and LSTM layers classify transitions like "walking → jogging."

Advantages of Automatic Feature Extraction

- Eliminates manual feature engineering
- Learns task-specific features end-to-end
- Scales better across subjects and datasets
- Improves generalization across activity contexts.

Step-by-step feature extraction method of HAR dataset using deep learning models is shown in Fig. 4.1.

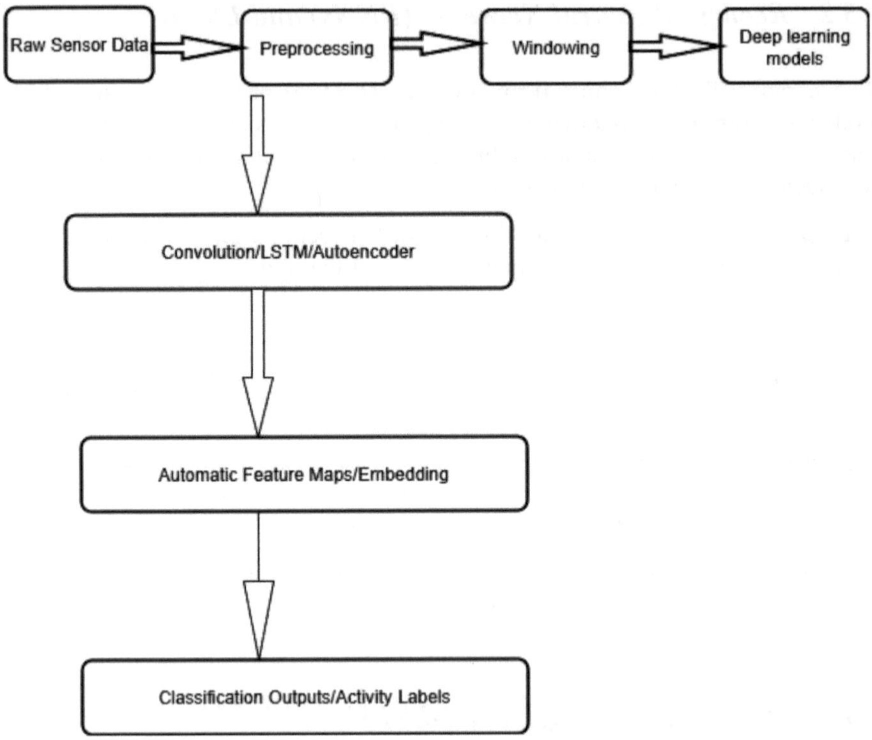

Fig. 4.1 Step-by-step feature extraction of HAR dataset using deep learning

4.6 Conclusion

Human activity recognition (HAR) stands at the forefront of innovation in ubiquitous computing, enabling machines to perceive and interpret human behaviors through sensor-based data. As demonstrated in this study, the integration of advanced machine learning techniques—particularly deep learning models such as convolutional neural networks (CNNs), recurrent neural networks (RNNs), and long short-term memory (LSTM) architectures—has transformed traditional approaches to activity recognition. These methods have proven to be powerful in capturing spatial and temporal patterns from multivariate time-series data collected via accelerometers, gyroscopes, and other wearable sensors.

The application of CNNs enables effective extraction of local spatial features, making them suitable for processing raw sensor signals without the need for extensive manual feature engineering. RNNs and their variants, such as LSTM and GRU, offer capabilities for learning from sequential dependencies, which are essential for capturing the dynamic nature of human movements over time. Combining CNN and RNN models further enhances the performance of HAR systems by leveraging the strengths of both architectures—CNNs for spatial encoding and RNNs for temporal sequencing. As a result, hybrid deep learning architectures have shown improved accuracy, generalization, and robustness in recognizing complex activity patterns. In conclusion, this study underscores the transformative impact of deep learning on the landscape of human activity recognition. By continuing to refine model architectures, address data and deployment challenges, and pursue interdisciplinary integration, HAR can evolve into a cornerstone technology for smart health care, assisted living, and intelligent human–machine interaction.

References

1. Bulling, A., Blanke, U., & Schiele, B. (2014). A tutorial on human activity recognition using body-worn inertial sensors. *ACM Computing Surveys, 46*(3), 1–33. https://doi.org/10.1145/2499621
2. Chen, Y., Shen, C., & Chen, C. (2020). A deep learning approach to activity recognition for post-stroke rehabilitation. *Sensors, 20*(5), 1416. https://doi.org/10.3390/s20051416
3. Ordóñez, F. J., & Roggen, D. (2016). Deep convolutional and LSTM recurrent neural networks for multimodal wearable activity recognition. *Sensors, 16*(1), 115. https://doi.org/10.3390/s16010115
4. Wang, J., Chen, Y., Hao, S., Peng, X., & Hu, L. (2019). Deep learning for sensor-based activity recognition: A survey. *Pattern Recognition Letters, 119*, 3–11. https://doi.org/10.1016/j.patrec.2018.02.010
5. Zeng, W., Zhou, X., Liu, X., & Wang, Y. (2021). Parkinson's disease detection using wearable sensor data and deep learning. *Frontiers in Aging Neuroscience, 13*, 629370. https://doi.org/10.3389/fnagi.2021.629370
6. Mallik, S., Majhi, B., Kashyap, A., Mohanty, S., Dash, S., Li, A., & Zhao, Z. (2022). An ensemble of CNN models for Parkinson's disease detection using DaTscan images. *BMC Medical Imaging, 22*(1), 1–12.
7. https://www.who.int/news-room/fact-sheets/detail/cardiovascular-diseases-(cvds)
8. Guan, R., & Plötz, T. (2017). Ensembles of deep LSTM learners for activity recognition using wearables. In *Proceedings of the ACM International Symposium on Wearable Computers* (pp. 11–18).
9. Zeng, M., Nguyen, L. T., Yu, B., Mengshoel, O. J., Zhu, J., Wu, P., & Zhang, J. (2014). Convolutional neural networks for human activity recognition using mobile sensors. In *Proceedings of the 6th International Conference on Mobile Computing, Applications and Services* (pp. 197–205).
10. Yang, J., Nguyen, M. N., San, P. P., Li, X., & Krishnaswamy, S. (2015). Deep convolutional neural networks on multichannel time series for human activity recognition. In *Proceedings of the 24th International Conference on Artificial Intelligence* (pp. 3995–4001).
11. Ha, S., Yun, J., & Choi, S. (2015). Multi-modal convolutional neural networks for activity recognition. In *Proceedings of the 2015 IEEE International Conference on Systems, Man, and Cybernetics* (pp. 3017–3022).
12. Carfi, A., Motolese, C., & Bruno, B. (2018). *Online human gesture recognition using recurrent neural networks and wearable sensors*. arXiv preprint arXiv:1810.11297. https://arxiv.org/abs/1810.11297
13. Lee, S., & Kim, J. (2021). Human activity recognition using 2D pose estimation and CNNs for healthcare monitoring. *IEEE Sensors Journal, 21*(3), 3482–3491.
14. Chen, Y., Xue, Y., & Shi, Y. (2020). Residual CNN for sensor-based human activity recognition in smart healthcare. *Sensors, 20*(4), 1075.
15. Ignatov, A., Radu, V., & Lane, N. D. (2018). Multi-head CNN-RNN for multimodal human activity recognition. *Information Fusion, 49*, 1–10.

16. Nweke, H. F., Teh, Y. W., Al-Garadi, M. A., & Alo, U. R. (2018). Deep learning algorithms for human activity recognition using mobile and wearable sensor networks: State of the art and research challenges. *Expert Systems with Applications, 105*, 233–261.
17. Sahoo, S. P., Ari, S., Mahapatra, K., & Mohanty, S. P. (2020). HAR-depth: A novel framework for human action recognition using sequential learning and depth estimated history images. *IEEE Transactions on Emerging Topics in Computational Intelligence, 5*(5), 813–825.
18. Huang, X., Yuan, Y., Chang, C., Gao, Y., Zheng, C., & Yan, L. (2023). Human activity recognition method based on edge computing-assisted and GRU deep learning network. *Applied Sciences, 13*(16), 9059. https://doi.org/10.3390/app13169059
19. Arokiaraj, S., & Viswanathan, N. (2023). ECG-NETS: A novel integration of capsule networks and extreme gated recurrent neural network for IoT-based human activity recognition. *Journal of Intelligent & Fuzzy Systems, 44*(5), 8219–8229. https://doi.org/10.3233/JIFS-221551
20. Singh, D., Jain, S., Arora, S., & Sangwan, S. (2020). *Deep ConvLSTM with self-attention for human activity decoding using wearables*. arXiv preprint arXiv:2005.00698. https://arxiv.org/abs/2005.00698
21. Lwanga, D., Wang, Y., & Han, X. (2023). Using a hybrid neural network and a regularized extreme learning machine for human activity recognition with smartphone and smartwatch. *Sensors, 23*(6), 3354. https://doi.org/10.3390/s23063354
22. Chen, Z., Wang, C., Wu, C., Wang, H., & Yu, L. (2021). An information gain-based model and an attention-based RNN for wearable human activity recognition. *Entropy, 23*(12), 1635. https://doi.org/10.3390/e23121635
23. Mekruksavanich, S., & Jitpattanakul, A. (2021). LSTM networks using smartphone data for sensor-based human activity recognition in smart homes. *Sensors, 21*(5), 1636. https://doi.org/10.3390/s21051636
24. Arora, G., Ahlawat, A., & Payal, M. (2021). Long short-term memory network for recognition of daily human activity. In *Proceedings of the 2nd International Conference on ICT for Digital, Smart, and Sustainable Development* (pp. 1–6).
25. Zhong, J., Liu, Y., Cheng, X., Cai, L., Cui, W., & Hai, D. (2022). Gated recurrent unit network for psychological stress classification using electrocardiograms from wearable devices. *Sensors, 22*(22), 8664. https://doi.org/10.3390/s22228664
26. Pan, J., Hu, Z., Yin, S., & Li, M. (2022). GRU with dual attentions for sensor-based human activity recognition. *Electronics, 11*(11), 1797. https://doi.org/10.3390/electronics11111797
27. Gao, W., Zhang, L., Teng, Q., He, J., & Wu, H. (2021). Multimodal attention networks for human activity recognition from wearable sensor data. *Proceedings of the ACM on Interactive, Mobile, Wearable and Ubiquitous Technologies, 5*(4), 1–23. https://doi.org/10.1145/3544793.3563422
28. Hossain, M. S., et al. (2021). HF-SPHR: Hybrid features for sustainable physical healthcare pattern recognition using deep belief networks. *Sustainability, 13*(4), 1699. https://doi.org/10.3390/su13041699
29. Jahanjoo, A., Naderan, M., & Rashti, M. J. (2020). Detection and multi-class classification of falling in elderly people by deep belief network algorithms. *Journal of Ambient Intelligence and Humanized Computing, 11*, 4145–4165. https://doi.org/10.1007/s12652-020-01690-z
30. Dhiravidachelvi, E., et al. (2023). Intelligent deep learning enabled human activity recognition for improved medical services. *Computer Systems Science & Engineering, 44*(2), 48246. https://doi.org/10.32604/csse.2023.024612
31. Kumar, P. A., et al. (2022). Fuzzy dragon deep belief neural network for activity recognition using hierarchical skeleton features. *Evolutionary Intelligence, 15*, 907–924. https://doi.org/10.1007/s12065-019-00245-2
32. Wang, J., et al. (2016). Human activity recognition using deep belief networks with feature selection. *Sensors, 16*(6), 869. https://doi.org/10.3390/s16060869
33. Chen, Y., et al. (2019). Enhancing human activity recognition using deep belief networks and data augmentation techniques. *IEEE Access, 7*, 21836–21845. https://doi.org/10.1109/ACCESS.2019.2897985

34. Wang, L. (2016). Recognition of human activities using continuous autoencoders with wearable sensors. *Sensors, 16*(2), 189. https://doi.org/10.3390/s16020189
35. Zhang, Y., et al. (2020). Leveraging wearable sensors for human daily activity recognition with stacked denoising autoencoders. *Sensors, 20*(18), 5114. https://doi.org/10.3390/s20185114
36. Chahoushi, M., Nabati, M., Asvadi, R., & Ghorashi, S. A. (2023). CSI-based human activity recognition using multi-input multi-output autoencoder and fine-tuning. *Sensors, 23*(7), 3591. https://doi.org/10.3390/s23073591
37. Alo, U. R., Nweke, H. F., Teh, Y. W., & Murtaza, G. (2020). Smartphone motion sensor-based complex human activity identification using deep stacked autoencoder algorithm for enhanced smart healthcare system. *Sensors, 20*(21), 6300. https://doi.org/10.3390/s20216300

Chapter 5
Machine Learning in Fall Detection Systems

5.1 Introduction

This section presents the core sensing mechanisms and data collection strategies that form the basis of human activity recognition (HAR) and fall detection (FD) systems. Accurate recognition depends on reliable sensor data that captures both motion and contextual cues related to human activities. The subsections introduce inertial measurement units (IMUs) as the primary sensors used to measure movement dynamics, including acceleration and angular velocity. Additional modalities such as load cells and pressure sensors offer valuable insight into balance and support-related behaviors, especially during pre-fall events. The final part emphasizes the importance of constructing well-labeled and diverse datasets—both public and custom-collected—to ensure that HAR/FD models perform reliably across various users, environments, and device placements.

5.1.1 Sensor Technologies and Data Acquisition

Sensor technologies have advanced rapidly in last few years and heterogeneous types of sensors sensing data in different format such as text, image, audio, and video. Some of these sensors being efficiently and majorly utilized in fall detection are described below.

5.1.1.1 Inertial Measurement Units (IMUs)

The cornerstone of most HAR/FD systems is the inertial measurement unit (IMU), which comprises a triaxial accelerometer and a triaxial gyroscope. These sensors measure linear acceleration (m/s^2) and angular velocity ($^\circ/s$), typically sampled at

S. Biswas, *Machine Learning and Deep Learning in Human Activity Recognition and Fall Detection*, Signals and Communication Technology,
https://doi.org/10.1007/978-3-032-09241-0_5

40–100 Hz to balance temporal resolution with power consumption. Raw data is first calibrated—correcting for sensor bias and scale factors—and then passed through a low-pass filter (e.g., a 4th-order Butterworth with a 20 Hz cutoff) to remove high-frequency noise. The SVM is defined as

$$\mathrm{SVM}(t) = \sqrt{a_x(t)^2 + a_y(t)^2 + a_z(t)^2}$$

It provides a single-dimensional representation of overall acceleration magnitude and highlights the high-impact spikes characteristic of falls [1]. Yet, SVM alone cannot distinguish a fall from similar dynamic activities, necessitating richer feature sets.

5.1.1.2 Load Cells, Pressure Sensors, and Auxiliary Modalities

To capture balance perturbations preceding a fall, advanced HAR systems embed load cells (e.g., YZC-133 with HX711 amplifier) into walking aids such as smart canes or quad-sticks. By measuring grip force distribution in Newtons, these devices detect sudden increases in applied force when a subject braces against instability [2, 3]. Noncontact infrared sensors (MLX90614) and ultrasonic rangefinders (HC-SR04) have also been used to monitor physiological parameters and user proximity in multimodal frameworks, although they lie beyond the primary scope of this chapter [4].

5.1.1.3 Dataset Construction

Robust ML models rely on diverse, well-labeled datasets. Public benchmarks include the UCI HAR dataset—recording six activities (walking, jogging, sitting, standing, upstairs, and downstairs) at 50 Hz from 30 subjects—and UMAFall, which captures standardized activities of daily living (ADLs) and falls using five body-worn nodes [4]. The KOA-PD-NM dataset further provides gait patterns for knee osteoarthritis, Parkinson's, and healthy controls [5]. To account for device placement variability and environmental conditions, research groups often collect complementary in-house data: 500-s smartphone trials at 40 Hz outdoors, with GPS fall localization tags, and trials on uneven terrain, enhancing model generalizability [1].

5.1.2 Preprocessing and Feature Extraction

This section outlines the procedures involved in transforming raw IMU data into a structured form suitable for activity recognition and fall detection. The process begins with filtering and segmenting the continuous sensor signals into fixed-length overlapping windows, typically 2 s long with 50% overlap. This segmentation helps preserve the temporal dynamics of human movement while making the data manageable for further analysis. Each window is then detrended and normalized to eliminate baseline drift and ensure uniformity across different recording sessions or devices.

5.1.2.1 Signal Filtering and Windowing

Once calibrated and denoised, continuous IMU streams are segmented into overlapping windows—commonly 2 s with 50% overlap—to preserve temporal continuity. Each window undergoes detrending, mean–variance normalization, and feature computation.

5.1.2.2 Time- and Frequency-Domain Features

Within each window, statistical features such as mean acceleration, standard deviation, root mean square (RMS), interquartile range, and zero-crossing rate capture signal dynamics. Frequency-domain features—dominant frequency, spectral entropy, and energy in designated bands via short-time Fourier transform—differentiate activities by their characteristic spectral signatures (e.g., walking peaks near 1.5 Hz, running near 3 Hz, and fall impacts above 10 Hz) [3].

5.2 Supervised Machine Learning for Activity Recognition

With well-structured features extracted from IMU signals, supervised machine learning offers a powerful approach to recognize and classify human activities. By learning patterns from labeled data, these models can effectively distinguish between various movements such as walking, running, sitting, or falling. The choice of classification algorithm and the strategy used to train and evaluate the model play a crucial role in determining the overall system performance. This section introduces the commonly used machine learning algorithms for activity recognition and outlines standard practices for model training, validation, and performance assessment.

5.2.1 Classification Algorithms

Machine learning classifiers commonly applied include support vector machines (SVM) with radial basis function kernels, random forest (RF) ensembles, k-nearest neighbors (k-NN), and increasingly, deep architectures such as one-dimensional convolutional neural networks (CNNs) and long short-term memory (LSTM) networks [2, 5]. RF offers robustness to noisy features and interpretable tree-based decisions, while CNNs automatically learn hierarchical temporal filters.

5.2.2 Model Training and Validation

Typical workflows allocate 70% of data for training, 15% for validation (hyperparameter tuning), and 15% for testing. K-fold cross-validation ($k = 5$) guards against overfitting. Performance is evaluated via accuracy, precision, recall, *F1*-score, and confusion matrices. RF classifiers often reach 95–98% accuracy on multiclass HAR tasks, whereas CNN-LSTM hybrids can exceed 98% on large datasets [3].

5.3 Fall Detection Architectures

Detecting falls in real time requires a careful balance between responsiveness, accuracy, and computational efficiency. As falls are often sudden and high-impact events, specialized architectural designs are necessary to ensure timely detection while minimizing false alarms. This section explores the key architectural strategies used in fall detection systems, ranging from simple threshold-based methods to more sophisticated hybrid and fully integrated solutions. Each approach reflects different trade-offs between local decision-making, communication overhead, and energy efficiency, offering insight into how fall detection can be effectively embedded into real-world wearable or IoT-based systems.

5.3.1 Threshold-Based Triggers

Low-latency on-device modules compute the SVM in real time, raising a fall candidate when SVM > 2.5 g within a window, and the post-impact SVM remains < 0.2 g for more than 1 s (stationarity check). This architecture ensures immediate response but can generate false positives under non-fall impacts [1].

5.3.2 Hybrid Threshold–ML Systems

To balance latency with accuracy, hybrid systems use an initial threshold check on the device to flag potential events and then transmit the buffered window to a server or fog node where an ML classifier (e.g., RF or SVM) confirms or rejects the event, dramatically reducing false alarms [1].

5.3.3 End-to-End System Integration

Embedded microcontrollers (ESP8266 or ESP32) package precomputed feature vectors and stream them using protocols such as MQTT to Raspberry Pi fog nodes or cloud platforms. Energy-efficient routing schemes based on two-state Markov mobility models adapt cluster-head election to network dynamics, improving packet delivery ratio (PDR) from 85% (LEACH-M) to 94% and reducing average energy consumption by 18% over 50 simulated rounds [6].

5.4 Fall Risk Analysis and Prediction

Beyond detecting falls as they occur, a critical aspect of proactive health care involves assessing an individual's likelihood of falling in the future [7]. Fall risk prediction aims to identify early signs of mobility impairment or instability, allowing for timely interventions before an actual incident takes place. This section introduces key methods used to evaluate fall risk, including standardized clinical assessments, biomechanical measurements, and data-driven models. By integrating multiple indicators—from timed mobility tasks to gait asymmetry and grip strength—modern systems can deliver comprehensive, personalized risk profiles that support preventive care and long-term monitoring.

5.4.1 Timed Up-and-Go (TUG) Test Metrics

The TUG test measures the time to rise from a chair, walk 5 m, turn, return, and sit. Clinical thresholds classify risk: < 10 s (low), 10–20 s (moderate), and > 20 s (high). Patients completing TUG in > 22 s often exhibit additional gait abnormalities warranting intervention [8, 9, 10]. Gait issues are prevalent in elderly people, and HAR can be applied for gait detection or gait symptoms prediction [11, 12].

5.4.2 Grip Force and Gait Symmetry

By monitoring grip force via load cells at 50 Hz, systems detect compensatory loading patterns. Gait symmetry index (GSI) defined as

$$\text{GSI} = \frac{\left|\text{stride\_time}_{\text{left}} - \text{stride\_time}_{\text{right}}\right|}{\text{mean}(\text{stride\_times})}$$

quantifies asymmetry; $\text{GSI} > 0.1$ correlates with freezing-of-gait and fall risk [5].

5.4.3 Multimodal Risk Models

Combining TUG time, average grip force flags, and GSI in logistic regression yields an ROC AUC of 0.93. Optimizing the decision threshold via Youden's index achieves 91% sensitivity and 88% specificity, enabling proactive risk stratification and personalized interventions [5].

5.5 System Evaluation and Benchmarking

To ensure reliability and generalizability, fall detection and activity recognition systems must be rigorously evaluated under diverse conditions and user populations. Benchmarking allows developers to compare models, end-to-end systems architectures, and deployment strategies using standardized datasets and well-defined performance metrics [13, 14]. This section outlines the key elements of system evaluation, including the datasets and testing protocols used, the metrics applied to quantify effectiveness, and comparative results that highlight the strengths and limitations of different approaches. Such evaluations are essential for validating system performance in real-world scenarios and guiding future improvements.

5.5.1 Datasets and Protocols

Models are benchmarked on public datasets (UCI HAR: $n = 30$; UMAFall: $n = 17$) and self-collected trials involving 40 volunteers aged 20–80, including 30 Parkinson's patients [1].

5.5.2 Performance Metrics

Evaluation metrics include true positive rate (TPR), false positive rate (FPR), precision, recall, $F1$-score, detection latency, PDR, and energy consumption per round [15].

5.5.3 Comparative Results

Table 5.1 summarizes prototype performance: smartphone FD (94.45% accuracy, 7.5% FPR), SWA fall/posture (98.0% accuracy, 4.2% FPR), fall-risk stick prediction (92.0% accuracy), and IoT network energy savings (18%) [1, 2, 5].

Table 5.1 Prototype performance metrics

System	Accuracy	False alarm rate	Latency (s)	Energy savings
Smartphone-based FD [1]	94.45%	7.5%	0.5	–
SWA fall/posture [2]	98.0%	4.2%	0.3	–
Risk analysis using walking stick [5]	92.0%	–	–	–
Hybrid IoT network [15]	–	–	–	18%

Visual representations and structured summaries play a crucial role in communicating system performance and design. This section presents key tables and figures that encapsulate experimental results and architectural layouts discussed in previous sections. The performance metrics table provides a comparative overview of different prototype systems, highlighting trade-offs in accuracy, false alarm rates, latency, and energy efficiency. The accompanying figures illustrate the core components and data flow of two representative implementations—a smartphone-based fall detection system and a sensor-embedded smart walking stick—offering a clear picture of how hardware and software elements integrate in practice.

Table 5.1 provides a comparative summary of the performance characteristics of four distinct prototype systems designed for fall detection and fall risk analysis. The smartphone-based fall detection system demonstrates high accuracy (94.45%) with moderate false alarm rates and low latency, making it suitable for real-time applications. The SWA fall/posture system achieves the highest accuracy (98.0%) and the lowest false alarm rate (4.2%), highlighting its effectiveness in discriminating between fall and non-fall events. The risk analysis using walking stick, though focused more on predictive assessment than immediate detection, still maintains a respectable accuracy of 92.0%. Finally, the hybrid IoT network, while not providing direct classification metrics, offers substantial energy savings (18%) through efficient data transmission and fog-based processing, which is crucial for long-term deployment in wearable and edge-based environments. Together, these results highlight the trade-offs among detection accuracy, system responsiveness, and energy efficiency in practical deployments.

Figure 5.1 illustrates the architecture of a threshold-based fall detection system implemented using a standard smartphone and a Raspberry Pi-based monitoring station. The smartphone, functioning as a sensor hub, continuously collects triaxial accelerometer data. When a potential fall is detected—characterized by high acceleration followed by prolonged inactivity—the system evaluates whether the user has self-recovered. If no recovery is detected, the system triggers a multistage response: an alert is generated locally, and a warning SMS is transmitted to predefined caregivers, including time and location of the incident. All processing and decision logic are offloaded to a Raspberry Pi 4, which supports Wi-Fi and Bluetooth, ensuring portability and real-time communication. Figure 5.1 outlines the data flow from sensing and fall detection to alert transmission, reflecting a cost-effective, low-latency, and socially acceptable solution particularly effective for Parkinson's patients, as validated in clinical trials.

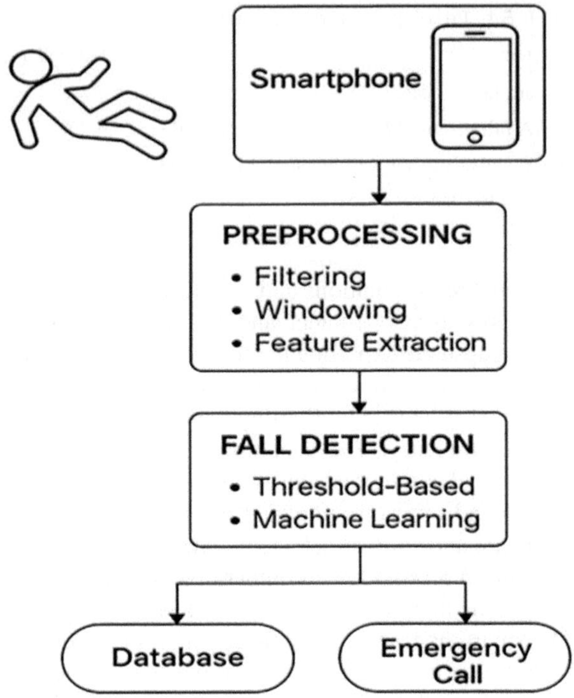

Fig. 5.1 Architecture of smartphone-based fall detection system [1]

Figure 5.2 shows the hardware prototype of a smart walking stick designed for real-time fall and posture detection. The system integrates an MPU6050 kinematic sensor (triaxial accelerometer and gyroscope) and a YZC-133 load cell amplified by an HX711 module to monitor both motion and grip force. These components are connected to an ESP8266 microcontroller that streams live sensor data over Wi-Fi to a Raspberry Pi-based fog server. The embedded system performs on-device fall detection using threshold-based analysis of signal vector magnitude (SVM), while posture recognition is handled server side using random forest classification. In the event of a fall without self-recovery, the system generates an audible-visual alert and sends an SMS to caregivers, including the subject's last known posture and location via Wi-Fi positioning. The prototype supports both manual (panic button) and automatic operation modes and has been tested across a wide age range, demonstrating high accuracy and energy-efficient performance. The figure also includes the circuit connections and a depiction of a user interacting with the device in a real-world scenario.

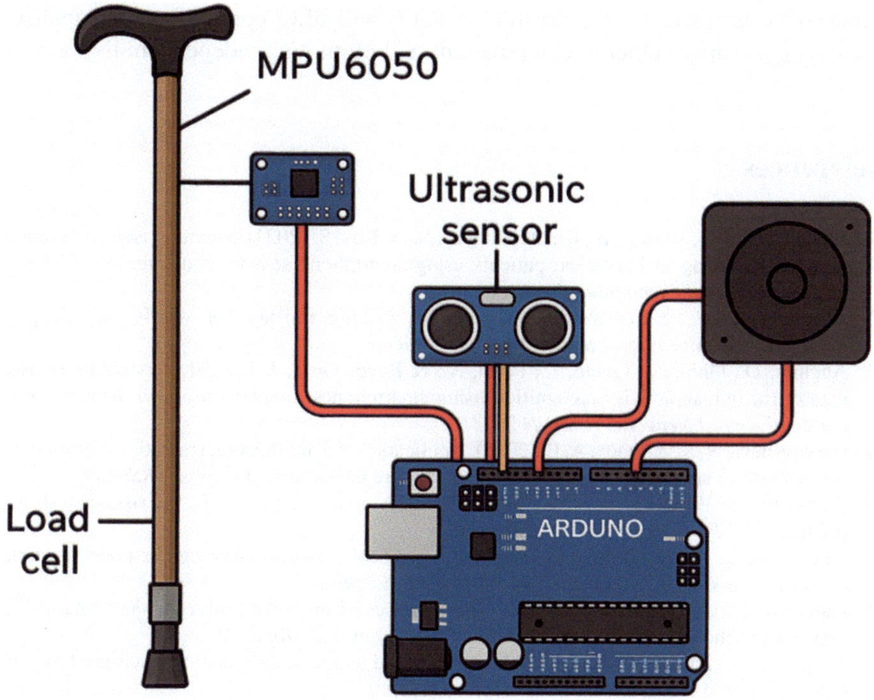

Fig. 5.2 Smart walking stick prototype with MPU6050 and load cell [2]

5.6 Challenges and Future Directions

Despite remarkable advances, HAR/FD systems face ongoing challenges in miniaturizing hardware without compromising battery life, developing algorithms that adapt to sensor orientation shifts, safeguarding user privacy in location-aware monitoring, and addressing data scarcity through federated and transfer learning. Future research should explore on-chip AI accelerators for real-time edge inference, domain adaptation to novel sensor modalities, and integration of physiological signals (ECG, EMG) for holistic risk assessment.

5.7 Conclusion

Machine learning has transformed HAR and FD from coarse threshold rules to nuanced, data-driven models that dramatically reduce false alarm rates and improve detection latency. Hybrid on-device and server-side architectures strike an optimal balance between responsiveness and accuracy, while multimodal risk models enable proactive fall-risk management. As wearable sensors, edge-AI, and secure IoT frameworks advance, next-generation systems will offer continuous, personalized care—safeguarding vulnerable populations and promoting independent living.

References

1. Bhattacharjee, P., Biswas, S., Chattopadhyay, S., & Roy, S. (2023). Smart assistance to reduce the fear of falling in Parkinson patients using smartphone sensors and Internet of Things. *Wireless Personal Communications.*
2. Bhattacharjee, P., & Biswas, S. (2021). Smart walking assistant for elderly care using an intelligent real-time hybrid model. *Evolving Systems.*
3. Anguita, D., Ghio, A., Oneto, L., Parra, X., & Reyes-Ortiz, J. L. (2013). A public domain dataset for human activity recognition using smartphones. In *21st European Symposium on Artificial Neural Networks (ESANN 2013).*
4. Chernysheva, N. S., & Ionov, A. B. (2015). Application of a multichannel radiation thermometer for increase in adequacy of non-contact temperature measurement results. *YRSNED.*
5. Bhattacharjee, P., Sarkar, I., & Biswas, S. (2025). A smart companion for fall risk analysis and prediction. *IEEE Internet of Things Journal.*
6. Tan, L., et al. (2020). Improved LEACH-M protocol for processing outlier nodes in aerial sensor networks. *IEICE Transactions on Communications.*
7. Gan, S.K.-E., & Yeo, J. Y. Y. (2020). The promises of microcontroller kits and smartphone apps for psychological research. *Scientific Phone apps and Mobile Device.*
8. Shajkofci, A. (2021). Correction of human forehead temperature variations measured by non-contact infrared thermometer. *IEEE Sensors Journal.*
9. Noor, Q., Taleb, A., & Walid, S. (2020). LEACH based protocols: A survey. *Advances in Science, Technology and Engineering Systems Journal.*
10. Azevedo, L. P., & Silva, M. V. L. (2021) Formal methods to analyze energy efficiency and security for IoT: A systematic review. *AINA.*
11. Wang Y, et al. (2022). The validity and reliability of a new intelligent three-dimensional gait analysis system in healthy subjects and patients with post-stroke. *Sensors.*
12. Aragaki, D. R., et al. (2009). Immediate effects of contralateral and ipsilateral cane use on normal adult gait. *PM&R.*
13. Bhattacharjee, P., Roy, S., Biswas, S., & Bose, R. (2022). Design of an energy-efficient probabilistic algorithm for a hybrid healthcare network. In *Proceedings of the International Conference on Communication, Devices and Computing.*
14. Nasr Esfahani, M., Shahgholi Ghahfarokhi, B., & Etemadi Borujeni, S. (2021). End-to-end privacy preserving scheme for IoT-based healthcare systems. *Wireless Networks, 27*(6), 4009–4037.
15. Saadeh, W., Butt, S. A., & Altaf, M. A. B. (2019). A patient-specific single sensor IoT-based wearable fall prediction and detection system. *IEEE Transactions on Neural Systems and Rehabilitation Engineering, 27*(5), 995–1003.

Chapter 6
Sensor Fusion-Based HAR for Disease Monitoring and Prediction

6.1 Introduction

Human activity recognition (HAR) based on sensors has received much attention in recent years [1, 2] due to the availability of advanced technologies (such as IoT, machine learning, and deep learning) and its important role in several applications (such as health monitoring, activities of daily living monitoring, fitness tracking, personalized health care, and early disease prediction [3]). The activity types and range could be huge—simple activities of daily living are static or dynamic such as sitting, standing, running, jumping, jogging, and lying. Whereas some are daily chores related such as cycling, biking, and climbing stairs up or down, and these are more complex. Further some activities are detailed life style-related activities such as ironing clothes washing utensils, eating food with fork at restaurant, and drinking water from a glass [4].

HAR-related research has observed immense growth in research in recent years with the use of ML, DL, etc. [5–7]. Single sensor-based HAR models are outdated nowadays because of external factors affecting model accuracy. Hence, utilizing different heterogeneous sensor data sensor fusion methods can accurately identify different types of activities applying different algorithms such as SVM, KNN, logistic regression, decision tree, Naïve Bayes, KNN, and ANN.

Sensor fusion is getting immense popularity because in this method, if one single sensor misses to capture any significant feature of a particular activity, the other sensor can capture that thus missing features contributing to the model accuracy will be stopped. Recent advancements in sensor fusion-based HAR show performance improvement justifying the need for it.

S. Biswas, *Machine Learning and Deep Learning in Human Activity Recognition and Fall Detection*, Signals and Communication Technology,
https://doi.org/10.1007/978-3-032-09241-0_6

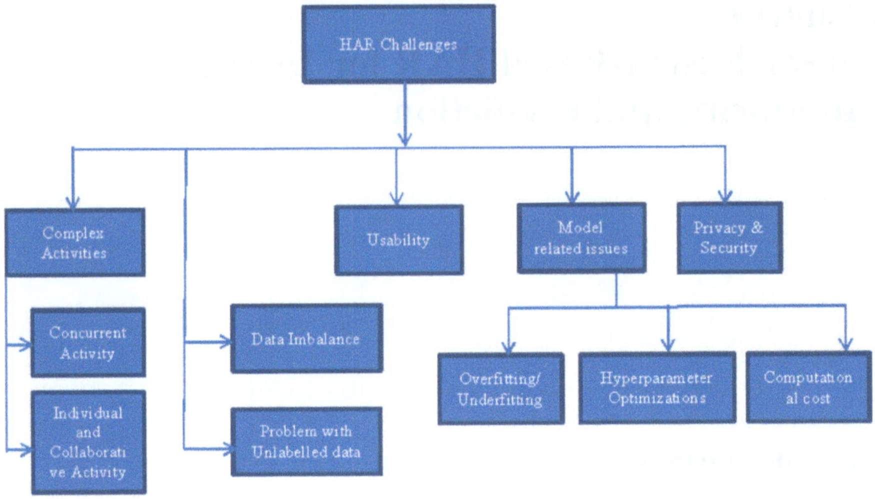

Fig. 6.1 Different information-fusion components and their working illustration

6.2 Challenges in HAR

There are various challenges in HAR as reported in the state-of-the-art literatures in recent times. And these challenged mainly are the driving factors behind the need of sensor fusion or multimodal data analysis for enhancing accuracy in human activity recognition which has immense real-time applications which are primarily dependent on the accuracy of the HAR system. Different challenges related to HAR are shown in Fig. 6.1. Major challenges are to identify complex activities and dataset-related issues, usability of the system is one of the major factor besides model performance-related matters, and obviously privacy and security issues as the HAR and FD-related raw sensory data carry sensitive information.

6.3 Information Fusion

When data gets generated from multiple type of sensors, smart devices need to be integrated for enhanced reliability, robustness, accuracy, validation and generalization purposes. Multi-sensor fusion is divided into three main categories:

i. Data-level fusion
ii. Feature-level fusion
iii. Decision-level fusion.

Information fusion is comprised of all three categories of fusion paradigms as mentioned above. Data fusion works with the principle of fusion of data from homogeneous or heterogeneous sensors. Irrespective of types of sensors, the working principle or basic steps of working are:

i. Sensor data collection
ii. Denoising
iii. Feature extraction
iv. Data classification
v. Data compression.

Scenario 1: Data collecting sensors are of same types—Homogeneous

The same physical signals or phenomenon collected from multiple similar types of sensors (homogeneous) can be fused directly, i.e., data fusion takes place directly with based working steps mentioned above.

Scenario 2: Data collecting sensors are of different types—Heterogeneous

Different sensor data collected through different types of sensors (heterogeneous) cannot be fused directly. Rather higher level fusion to be done, i.e., feature-level or decision-level fusion methodologies need to be applied.

Feature-level fusion

When direct data fusion is not feasible due to heterogeneity in sensor data, next level fusion that could be done is feature fusion. Now, what is the basic concept is to combine basic data features into high-dimensional feature vector to input to the classifier or pattern recognition process.

To combine different basic features extracted from sensors may be at different physical locations, different machine learning algorithms such as support vector machine (SVM), hidden Markov models (HMM), decision tree (DT), etc., can be used to distinctively analyze data at higher levels of abstraction.

Deep learning models such as CNN, ANN, and LSTM could be applied for automatic feature extraction, thus avoiding the issues related to spatial and temporal dependence problems.

Decision-level fusion

Hypothesis generated by individual decisions from multiple sensors are combined to generate a more unique, generalized hypothesis and is done in the decision-level fusion process.

6.4 Sensors in Sensor Fusion for Activity Recognition

6.4.1 Smartphone Sensors

Smartphone is sensor hub with more than 50 sensors in it. Various in-built sensors are being used in human activity recognition (HAR), e.g., accelerometer, gyroscope, magnetometer, etc. 3-axis accelerometer sensor is used to measure acceleration of the subject, gyroscope measures rotation which is very important to identify dynamic activities such as stairs up and stairs down, magnetometer measures orientation, GPS sensor provides location of the concerned one, and barometer can be used to measure altitude changes.

6.4.1.1 Accelerometer in HAR

An **accelerometer** is a sensor that measures **acceleration forces**—both from movement (kinetic) and gravity. It typically records acceleration in **three axes (*X*, *Y*, and Z)**. As an individual moves, the accelerometer captures variations in velocity over time on the X, Y, and Z axes. For instance: Walking generates regular, moderate-amplitude fluctuations. Running exhibits a greater frequency and amplitude. Sitting or standing displays minimal changes.

6.4.2 Feature Extraction

Raw acceleration data is processed into features such as:

- Mean, standard deviation, energy, and entropy
- Signal magnitude area (SMA)
- Fourier Transform features (frequency analysis).

6.4.3 Classification

These features are fed into machine learning models (like SVM, random forest, or neural networks) to classify the activity:

Examples: walking, running, standing, sitting, climbing stairs, cycling.

Few applications developed using accelerometer sensors:

1. Activity and fall monitoring of elderly
2. Estimating metabolic energy expenditure during exercise
3. To ensure improved quality of patient care

4. Gait parameters measurement, gait detection.

6.4.4 Advantages of Accelerometers in HAR

Accelerometer is preferred in many of the state-of-the-art literatures for mainly following advantages:

i. It ensures low power consumption already embedded in smartphones and wearable
ii. Reliable motion data
iii. Can work in real time
iv. Easy to integrate with existing sensor-based development.
v. Can display human motion changes with respect to motion frequency, tilt, and intensity and hence shows better performance in case of static postures.

Accelerometer alone may not be able to recognize activities with satisfactory accuracy in cases of dynamic, complex, composite, and fine grain posture detection, and hence, multimodal sensor fusion may be required. In various works, it has been reported with experimental results that when accelerometer sensor data has been combined with other inertial sensor, i.e., gyroscope, physiological sensor, e.g., ECG sensor, microphone, etc., for providing more useful information. In-spite of various advantages of accelerometer sensor, it needs to be combined with heterogeneous sensors to develop applications for all sorts of activities such as zero displacement activities, transitional activities, activities related to daily household cores or lifestyle activities may be at restaurants or shopping malls, strong dynamic activities due to physical fitness training at gym or park, etc. In these dynamic types of activities along with motion, tilt, intensity etc., direction of motion is very much important, and gyroscope which is an inertial sensor performs best in direction estimation of human motion or movement or activity.

6.4.5 Why Accelerometer and Gyroscope give better Performance when Combined?

Accelerometer measures both static force, i.e., gravity and dynamic force, i.e., vibration or movement during acceleration that acts on the sensor, thus helping in recognizing movement patterns. 3-axis accelerometer records the linear acceleration of three orthogonal axes: along x-axis horizontal acceleration, forward acceleration along y-axis, and the z-axis measures vertical acceleration. Accelerometer as single source of motion data is not sufficiently capable of identifying similar pattern of dynamic activities such as stairs up or stairs down.

On the other hand, gyroscope can measure the angular velocity during human movement, i.e., the rate of change of orientation of the motion sensor during dynamic

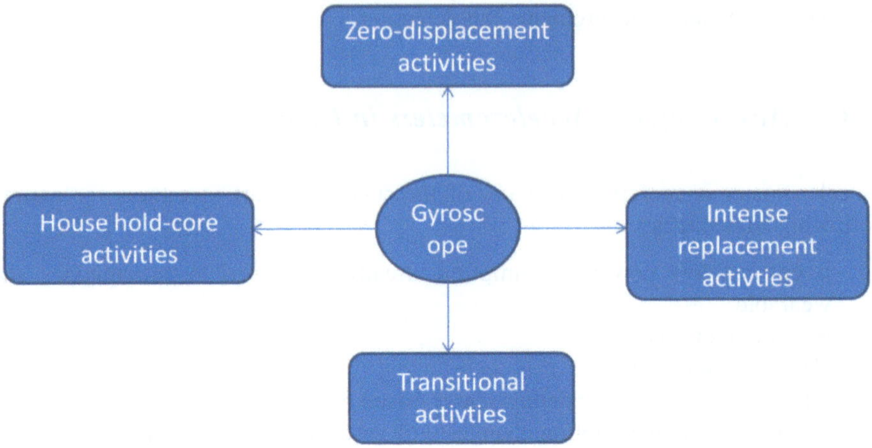

Fig. 6.2 Application of gyroscope in recognition of different activities

activity that causes rotation around a particular axis, and thus, dynamic activity pattern gets recognized by the gyroscope sensor. Figure 6.2 illustrates utilities of gyroscope sensor useful in dynamic human activity recognition. Accelerometer and gyroscope sensors complement each other and ensure improved accuracy in HAR, and thus when combined together in a single device, then they are called inertial measuring unit (IMU). Gyroscope measures the angular acceleration from three different angles, i.e., pitch, roll, and yaw, and this helps to estimate the orientation and rotation of the movement being captured.

6.5 Data Fusion

The process to gather data using multiple sources (sensors here) may be same type or different type for detailed insight, analysis, and pattern generation of specific information in comparison with using single source is called data fusion. Figure 6.3 gives representation of data fusion process that combines or refers to sensory data from multiple sensors to train the model for specific pattern identification.

6.5.1 Example of Data Fusion Using IMU Sensors in HAR

Accelerometer and gyroscope both are IMU sensors may be in wearable form or embedded in a smartphone and are widely used in human activity recognition as a single source or unit for human movement pattern recognition with enhanced accuracy. Accelerometer records linear acceleration, and the gyroscope sensors record

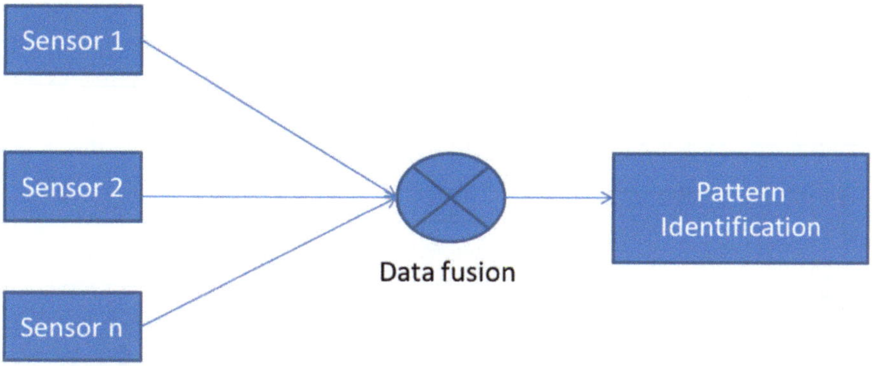

Fig. 6.3 Data fusion using multiple sensors for pattern identification with enhanced accuracy

angular velocity of the same human activity, motion, or movement. Combined these two sensors together can better be performing the utilization of gathered information to improve knowledge gathering on accurate position, orientation, or velocity of a subject or an object in concern.

Fusion of information gathered by different sensors immediately after data sensing and before feature extraction is called data fusion or sensor fusion.

Features are attributes of human motion or movement gathered by accelerometer and gyroscope sensors, and these can be divided into different categories such as time domain features, frequency domain features, or in wavelet domain.

For decision or accuracy enhancement, multiple models or classifiers are applied on same data to find different level of accuracy, precision, recall, etc. Decision-level fusion enhances performances of weak classifiers by combining their individual outputs to a more accurate classification. Now among these three types of fusion techniques, which one is most suitable in HAR is a research question which has been explored by different state-of-the literatures [5]. Figure 6.4 shows different levels of fusion methods and how they are utilized to achieve human activity recognition with enhanced security.

6.5.2 Sensor Fusion

The most basic fusion is sensor-level fusion among the three different fusion-level types as discussed earlier and is based on mostly signal processing techniques. Different filters are used in **HAR using IMU sensors**, to fuse various sensor data with noise such as accelerometer, gyroscope signals to get HAR and FD results with enhanced accuracy and reliability. These filters are applied to reduce noise and estimate orientation and smoothing signals. Table 6.1 shows different filters, their functions, system where these filters have been applied, and corresponding sensors used.

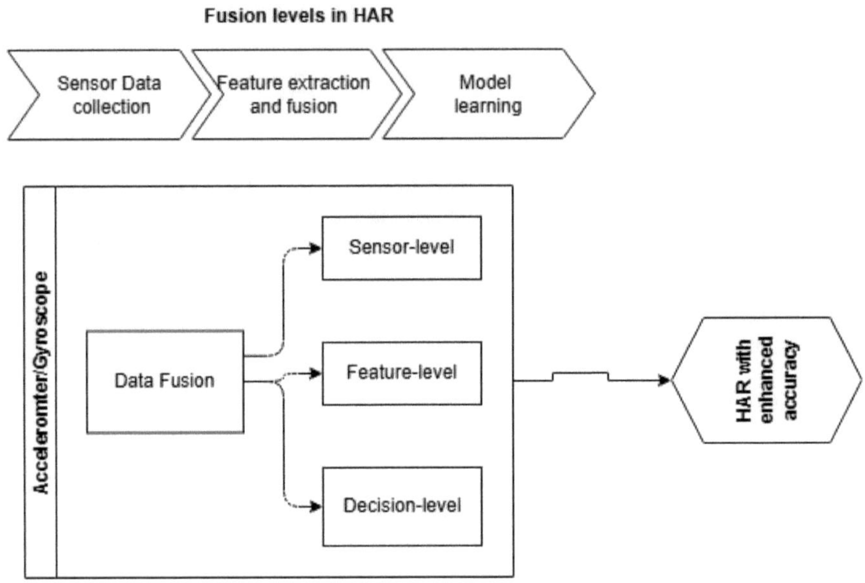

Fig. 6.4 Different fusion levels in HAR using IMU sensors

Table 6.1 Different filters used in sensor fusion

	Function	Applications developed	Sensor used
Kalman filter	Determines state of the subject under movement or motion	(i) Gait issues (ii) Parkinson's disease patients' postural analysis for behavioral monitoring (iii) Ambulatory movement analysis	Accelerometer and gyroscope, sensors fusion
Complementary filter	Removes unnecessary spikes in accelerometer signal and drift in gyroscope data using high-pass filter and low-pass filter	(i) Human movement recognition (ii) Gait analysis	Accelerometer and gyroscope, sensors fusion
Signal magnitude vector (SMV) and absolute vertical acceleration (AVA)	Removal of noise from accelerometer signal and reduces drift in angular velocity	Accident detection Movement monitoring Fall detection	Accelerometer and gyroscope, sensors fusion

6.5.2.1 Fusion at Feature Level

In data fusion or sensor-level fusion, first raw signals for multiple sensing sources are combined, and then, next necessary steps are performed for HAR and fall detection. Unlikely, in feature-level fusion, attributes of different signals sensed by multiple sources are combined before being fed to machine learning algorithms. Now it may come in mind, why fusion at feature level is required or what might be its significance from the point of view of performance improvement in HAR and fall detection applications? The answer lies to the fact that attributes or properties of signals captured by multiple sources either may be highly correlated, i.e., redundant features carrying similar information and may be removed, or may not be much relevant, i.e., features with low variance, hence also may be removed. So, these techniques after feature fusion actually ensures reduce number of features by which HAR can be performed with enhanced accuracy. And as number of features used is less, computation complexity, computation time, storage, etc., also get reduced, thus making these methodology-based applications more suitable for mobile and wearable sensor-based systems.

6.5.2.2 Methods Applied in Feature-Level Fusion

Mainly two types of feature-level fusion methods are applied:

i. Feature selection
ii. Dimensionality reduction.

Both of these techniques reduce total number of features using which HAR will be performed, and only basic difference lies in the working principle applied in both the methods. Feature selection actually reduces dimension by the method applied is to eliminate irrelevant or highly correlated features and creates a subset of effective features from original feature set. On the other hand, dimensionality reduction methods devise new features by fusing actual features from the feature set. Some popular and efficient dimensionality reduction techniques are: (i) Principle component analysis (PCA), (ii) Multidimensional scaling (MDS), (iii) Singular value decomposition (SVD), and (iv) Factor analysis (FA). These methods are well experimented and utilized to fuse features of accelerometer and gyroscope data in various applications on HAR, FD, etc.

6.5.2.3 Decision-Level Fusion

Now, once we are familiar with the methods and purpose of data fusion and feature fusion, question that arises in our mind is what is the need of decision-level fusion? What is done in decision-level fusion and what are the different methodologies or techniques being applied in state-of-the-art HARliteratures? The answer remains in the performance improvement scope of a single classifier or learning model while fusing multiple intermediate classifiers' outputs toward final decision. This performance improvement scope while multiple classifiers' outputs are fused in compared to a single classifier's performance while used in isolation lies to the facts that a single or individual classifier may performance poor in case of imbalanced dataset, large dataset, dataset with outliers, missing data, redundant data, high-dimensional data or lack of appropriate training data, etc. Popular and efficient methodologies of decision-level fusion are bagging, boosting, stacking, majority voting, etc. In ensemble bagging method, individual classifiers work on a nonoverlapping chunk of data from the whole, large dataset, and then outputs of individual classifiers are combined to find the improved result. These bagging, boosting, stacking, and majority voting techniques are well applied in various HAR applications [6].

Multiple sensor fusion methods as discussed above in detail are presented in Fig. 6.5 showing different processing steps involved in data fusion, feature fusion, and decision-level fusion methods.

6.6 Sensors Used in Various Fusion Methods for HAR, Fall Detection, and Healthcare Applications

6.6.1 Sensors in HAR and Fall Detection

6.6.1.1 Inertial Sensors

Mostly used inertial sensors are accelerometer, gyroscope, magnetometer, etc., for various HAR and FD applications for monitoring and healthcare purposes. Purpose could be activity or posture detection, fall detection, gait detection, fitness tracking, patient monitoring, etc. A real-time application has been developed by attaching inertial motion sensors on gloves so that the direction of wheel could be estimated to find the pressure level of the person behind the wheels, i.e., driver, and this work is reported in [7].

6.6.1.2 Physiological Sensors

Parallel to wide utilization of inertial sensors for HAR and fall detection, physiological sensors are also used for similar applications specifically for HAR. Physiological sensors used commonly are electrocardiogram (ECG), electroencephalogram (EEG), electromyography (EMG) sensors, etc. How these physiological sensors can help in HAR? Take the instance of ECG sensor signals captured of a person during different activities or exercise. The features that are extracted from the ECG signals are R-peaks or systolic peaks, maximum slopes, onset of PPG, etc., morphological features. Now, inertial sensor data fusion with ECG sensor data helps in finding variation in different morphological features during different activities, specifically in

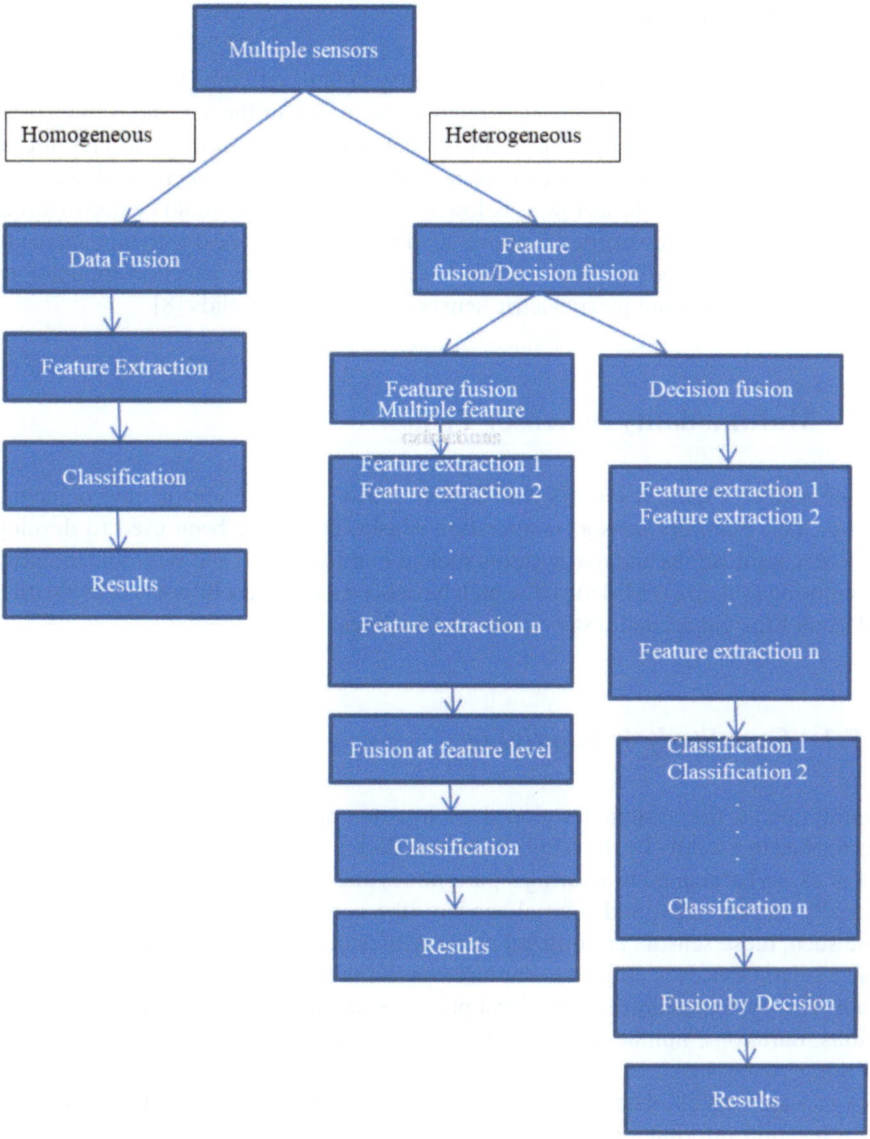

Fig. 6.5 Total fusion methodology description

high intense activities, activities performed carrying some weight like weight training at gymnasium, etc.

6.6.1.3 Pressure Sensors

Pressure sensor variants can be used to identify human activities based on the level of pressure exerted on the sensors through performance of the specific activity. The activity could be squatting which can be identified by measuring the pressure at knee joint where pressure sensor can be mounted while performing the activity. Also pressure exerted could be as low as below 100 Pa, and then, it would be due to throat vibration, or if pressure exerted is above 20 kPa, then it could be due to high intensity exercise such as squatting. Some sensor-based eye movement detection applications are also designed using piezoelectric sensors mounted on eyelids [8].

6.7 Multimodality in Sensor Fusion

Combination of inertial sensors with camera sensor, acoustic sensor, environmental sensor, i.e., humidity sensor, temperature sensor, etc., have been used to develop different applications and real systems such as FamilyLog [9] and wearable mobility monitoring system (WMMS) [10] which have been used as useful tools in evaluating different lifestyle-related observations and findings.

6.7.1 Case Study 1: FamilyLog

FamilyLog is the system developed to monitor and analyze different activities performed in a family by the family members during meal time. As nowadays almost all of us are habituated in wearing smartphones and smartwatches, these devices are actually sensor hubs, and inertial sensors like accelerometer and gyroscopes are one such, these sensors are utilized along with acoustic sensor, i.e., microphone of these smart devices is utilized to capture conversation, TV sounds, etc., during meal time. This system analyzes behavioral practices of a family during meal times, their habits, durations, number of members participating in meals together, their habit of doing discussions, or just taking meal only, no conversations, or habitual practice of watching TV, listening to music, etc. Also, if GPS sensor could be included, then location information also could be included to find a pattern of taking meals at outside eateries or invitation or parties as well, and these give lifestyle-related behavioral patterns. Date, time, and location add extra information about meal times which are at fixed hour of the day or vary over a small time range or a wide time range just to have a pattern analysis which can reveal the changing pattern indicating to lifestyle issues affecting meal-taking pattern in a family. And these would be giving better accuracy due to sensor fusion using multimodal data capture and analysis.

6.7.2 *Case Study 2: WMMS*

Combining inertial sensors and vision base sensors along with GPS and timer, this wearable mobility monitoring system is applied to capture data and analyze and identify mobility changes during change of one activity to another (static), during household chores like cooking, working in kitchen, etc.

Concurrent human activities recognition using multilocation sensor fusion:

Till now activities considered so far are single activity being performed at a particular time instance or duration. But in real life, during daily chores of life, it is quite common to perform multiple activities at the same time, and these are called concurrent activities. The example of concurrent activities could be:

i. Eating and watching TV
ii. Walking and brushing teeth
iii. Walking and combing hair
iv. Cooking and listening to music
v. Sitting and painting
vi. Lying and talking over phone
vii. Standing and capturing photo or video.

Now the challenge is to identify these concurrent activities with higher accuracies. For that purpose, multiple inertial sensors such as accelerometer and gyroscope are being used at different position of human body based on the types of activities.

Based on the activities performed and variation in pressure exerted on inertial sensors according to their positions on the human body, different sensors give varying levels of accuracies for the same activity. During simple activities such as sleeping accelerometer sensor at wrist will give higher accuracy, whereas during dynamic activities such as walking, running, and jogging, ankle and knee sensors would give better accuracy, etc.

Figure 6.6 depicts the processing and differentiation between two different methodologies between machine learning and deep learning algorithms. The main difference is in feature extraction method, and based on the type, dimensionality, type, and complexity of dataset, deep learning is preferred over machine learning as it provides automatic feature extraction compared to handcrafted feature extraction in HAR.

6.8 Conclusion

Finally we come to the observation that in order to address the issues of using one sensor and improve the performance of the recognition, researchers have proposed methods of multi-sensor data fusion. Using multiple sensors for recognizing human activities performs better because the information not recorded by one sensor can

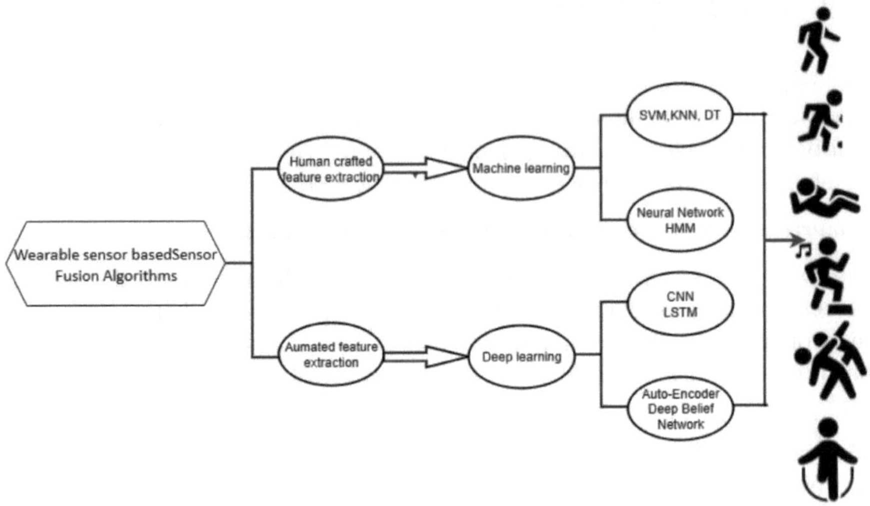

Fig. 6.6 Multimodal sensor fusion-based algorithms for HAR

be supplied by other sensors. And the level of accuracy and precision will obviously improve. State-of-the-art research works have presented accuracy improvement with sensor fusion using multiple sensors in comparison with single sensor. There are plenty of methods to combine the information acquired from several similar or different sensors, and there are active research areas called data fusion, sensor fusion, information fusion, etc. Even when restricting our attention to multi-sensor fusion in the context of HAR and fall detection, there are hundreds of specific works having used many variants of combinations of fusion methods, and each author claims to have achieved better results than others, so the need for putting some order in this area seems evident.

References

1. Aarts, E., & Wichert, R. (2009). Ambient intelligence. In H. J. Bullinger (Ed.), *Technology guide* (pp. 244–249). Springer.
2. Ponce, H., Miralles-Pechuán, L., & Martínez-Villaseñor, M. D. L. (2016). A flexible approach for human activity recognition using artificial hydrocarbon networks. *Sensors, 16*, 1715.
3. Su, X., Tong, H., & Ji, P. (2014). Activity recognition with smartphone sensors. *Tsinghua Science and Technology, 19*, 235–249.
4. Huynh, T., Fritz, M., & Schiele, B. (2008). Discovery of activity patterns using topic models. In *Proceedings of the 10th International Conference on Ubiquitous Computing*, Seoul, Korea, September 21–24, 2008 (pp. 10–19).
5. Webber, M., & Rojas, R. F. (2021). Human activity recognition with accelerometer and gyroscope: A data fusion approach. *IEEE Sensors Journal, 21*(15), 16979–16989.

6. Nweke, H. F., et al. (2019). Data fusion and multiple classifier systems for human activity detection and health monitoring: Review and open research directions. *Information Fusion Journal, 64*, 147–170.
7. Lee, B. G. (2016). Wearable glove type driver stress detection using a motion sensor. *IEEE Transaction on Intel Transportation System, 18*(7), 1835–1844.
8. Rigas, L., & Raffle, H. (2017). Hybrid ps-v technique: A novel sensor fusion approach for fast mobile eye-tracking with sensor-shift aware correction. *IEEE sensor Journal, 17*(24), 8356–8366.
9. Lara, O. D., & Labrador, M. A. (2013). A survey on human activity recognition using wearable sensors. *IEEE Communications Surveys & Tutorials, 15*(3), 1192–1209. https://doi.org/10.1109/SURV.2012.110112.00192
10. Ordóñez, F. J., & Roggen, D. (2016). Deep convolutional and LSTM recurrent neural networks for multimodal wearable activity recognition. *Sensors, 16*(1), 115. https://doi.org/10.3390/s16010115

Chapter 7
Design and Prototypes of HAR and FD Systems

7.1 Introduction

First of all, any design, development, and deployment begin with data collection or capturing or gathering, and here the data-capturing elements are mainly sensors. Now if we look at evolution history of HAR, the sensors used for raw data collection were primarily IMU sensors in wearable form, i.e., accelerometer or gyroscope. And also another type of input data collection devices used primarily has been camera sensors, then CCTV cameras installed in strategic positions at indoor or at outdoor, thus enabling HAR and FD at both the places without any movement area restrictions. Also in this later system, the user or the subject need not to be bothered about his or her involvement in data collection or generation, rather he or she in free to move, and knowingly or unknowingly the person is contributing in data gathering [1].

Also, initial methods or systems have been designed and developed to handle with homogeneous type of sensors gathering homogeneous data and that could be either text, image, numeric values, videos, etc. Applying threshold-based approached or applying supervised machine learning algorithms such as SVM, DT, NB, and KNN on single modal data, accuracy of HAR and FD systems in real time was not giving very good level of accuracy.

With the development of embedded technologies, availability of tiny, lightweight, affordable different types of sensors such as physiological sensors, pressure sensor, environmental sensors, piezoelectric sensors, and acoustic sensors, combining inertial sensors with one or more of other sensory data the practical systems being developed nowadays as are utilizing multimodal data. Hence, data size, data complexity, and volume all are increasing. To handle with such huge dataset, single, base machine learning-based classifiers such as SVM and KNN are not sufficient to give higher accuracy.

S. Biswas, *Machine Learning and Deep Learning in Human Activity Recognition and Fall Detection*, Signals and Communication Technology,
https://doi.org/10.1007/978-3-032-09241-0_7

7.1.1 *Using Sensor, IoT, and Cloud—Most Popularly Explored in HAR and FD for Health Care*

Also another factor or constraint or limitation is the miniaturization of computing devices while they are equipped with several other advantages such as mobility, portability, reliability, and efficiency. Sensors are mainly equipped with transceiver unit and actuation unit, and some of them are having microcontroller unit that can do some elementary data preprocessing such as noise elimination, filtering, and data redundancy check. So, sensors mainly just collected/gather/generate data and send to the processing unit through gateway. Now the gateway, sink, hub could be smartphones, tablet computers, routers, laptops, etc., having limited computing abilities, and these are called edge devices. These edge devices are having limited resources with limited computational abilities, and these are participatory devices in HAR or FD from the point of view of processing some emergency, time-critical data with higher priority. Many of the applications have been designed with data priority concept where time-critical systems and life-critical applications such as HAR and FD for heart patients utilizing accelerometer, gyroscope, ECG sensors, etc., in case of a fall event or if the person in doing high intensity exercises or activities, and if ECG signal shows some abnormal data, then the ECG signal packets need to be given high priority and should be analyzed first at edge end to identify the criticality of the person and generate alert push message in the doctor, hospital, or relative's registered mobile for immediate action. Or, in normal scenario, the raw data would be directly sent to the cloud server for storage, analysis, knowledge generation, and further giving access of information to the stakeholder for immediate legitimate action.

Now, while designing a system comprising of sensor, IoT, and cloud, the primary things that need to be taken care of are the stage at which the data needs to be stored and processed. Again, as the multimodal data for HAR and FD is big data in nature, resource-intensive complex models or algorithms need to be applied at which stage-at edge or at cloud? Now, the deciding factors could be many:

1. The dimension of dataset, complexity of the problem, and capability of the devices to be handle computations.
2. If the data is normal routine data or emergency, priority data?
3. If the data is processed at edge end—low latency, if the data is processed at cloud end—high latency: what the particular scenario is demanding or what the whole application is demanding?
4. If data is limited to edge end, the communication protocols or links through which data gets transmitted are short-range communication protocols like Wi-Fi, Bluetooth, etc. Whereas if data is sent to cloud end, data is sent through short-range and long-range communication protocols/links making the data being vulnerable to security attacks and threats that are prevalent in open wireless channels. So, privacy and security of data is a big concern.
5. Reliability, robustness, portability, usability, and affordability are the challenges that need to be taken care of at the system level that will be in practical use.

7.1.2 *Using Radar Technology for Health Care—Less Explored Pathway*

Radar technology is very commonly used in defense applications and very less explored in HAR and FD [2]. The reasons behind may be many, one of the very simple reason is that radar may not be available anywhere and everywhere covering daily activities and movements, and also it may be a costly affair compared to sensor-based HAR systems. Using RADAR technology, the subjects in concern can be monitored over wide region, and their whole body movements due to daily chores, exercises, different activities such as walking and running can be captured in proactive manner without bothering or directly involving them. Along with whole body movement, body part movements such as head, hand, or leg movements can also be captured and recognized. Moreover, very fine movements such as motions of the chest and abdomen while breathing, etc., could also be identified with accuracy. With this ability of identifying such very small-scale movements, the vital physiological parameters such as heart rate, pulse rate, and breathing rate could also be measured using RADAR technology. With all these abilities, RADAR is now being applied for HAR [3], FD, and healthcare applications by many of the organizations for both research purposes and in real-time practice. The other reasons of using RADAR technology which is increasing its popularity and applicability on HAR, FD, health monitoring, and healthcare applications are as follows:

i. A reliable approach for detecting the presence of individuals,
ii. Tracking movements of individuals within a certain coverage area or space
iii. Recognition of body or body parts movements
iv. Body parts movements could be large-scale movements such as head movement or limbs movement
v. To small-scale movements such as due to natural processes like breathing, motions of the chest and abdomen
vi. Such features of RADAR technology lead to its application not limited to defense applications only, rather spreading it out to detect or monitor everyday living activities like cooking, cleaning, gardening, etc.
vii. Monitoring activities or movements help in finding daily movement or activity pattern
viii. Any abnormality in daily activity or movement pattern may be identified, and alarm could be raised like in case of any sudden fall event occurs.

Now, whatever could be the data-gathering devices or systems, may be inertial sensors, camera sensors, drone camera or RADAR, the dataset is huge, and data analytics techniques need to be applied. In HAR and FD, popularly used models are applying advanced methodologies or algorithms such as artificial intelligence, deep learning, neural networks, reinforcement learning, GAN-based systems, CNN, LSTM, DNN, and ANN; accuracy level has been improved remarkably. There is scope of accuracy enhancement at different phases of human activity recognition. Now, while we apply these advanced AI-based models on multimodal data ranging over numeric, text, image, audio, video, physiological signals like ECG, EEG, EMG, etc., the concerns or the challenges that become prevalent are as follows:

1. Feasibility
2. Computational complexity
3. Computing system support
4. Computing decision either at edge or at cloud
5. Sensory data streaming, analysis, and result generation at real time
6. Time-critical applications
7. Priority data handling
8. System limitations
9. System performance
10. Privacy and security
11. Cost of development
12. Usability
13. Affordability
14. Portability
15. Flexibility.

There is always scope for performance improvement, so along with machine learning, deep learning algorithms, application of metaheuristic (MH) algorithms are also widely being used to address the challenge of handling high-dimensional data, thus reducing computational time, complexity, storage requirements, etc. As we all know, metaheuristic algorithms are utilized to optimize different complex computational problems. Here in HAR and FD-related research, MH algorithms are mostly applied to optimize selection of features so that accuracy boosting would be possible with reduces computational complexity and time. In [4], authors have applied different MH algorithms such as aqua optimizer (AO), marine predators algorithm (MPA), genetic algorithm (GA), arithmetic optimization algorithms (AOA), whale optimization algorithm (WOA), slime mold algorithm (SMA), grey wolf optimizer (GWO), particle swarm optimization (PSO), and artificial bee colony (ABC) have been used for feature selection purpose.

The basic steps followed for features selection before classification algorithms being applied are illustrated in the form of a flowchart as described in [5] which are as follows in Fig. 7.1. At the very beginning, the data preprocessing and segmentation methods are applied to find the pattern of movement or motion of the subject. Purpose of segmentation and preprocessing is also to reduce time complexities as well. Next step done has been development of a lightweight feature extraction technique applying advance deep learning approaches. They have developed the model called ResRNN that is comprised of several building blocks of multiple deep learning algorithms—convolutional neural network (CNN), bidirectional recurrent neural network (BiRNN), and residual network (ResNet). After all these computational processing, optimization algorithms, i.e., metaheuristics algorithms have been applied for selection of optimal features and to enhance or boosting of accuracy.

Feature optimization is a very significant process needs to be applied for multimodal complex large size HAR datasets having a huge number of features. MH

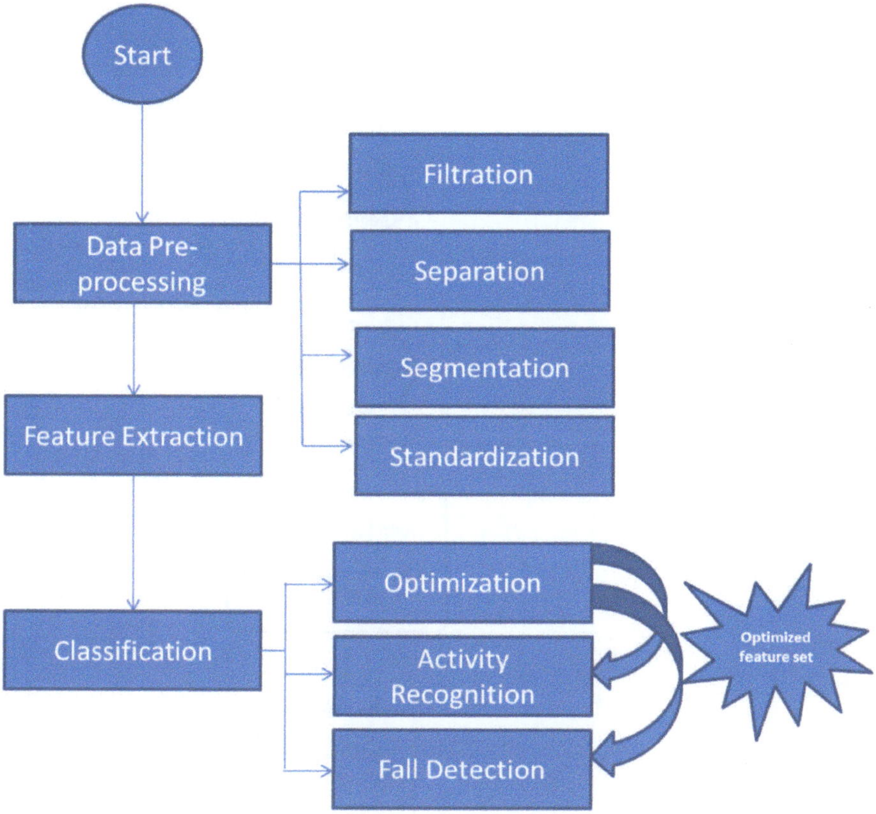

Fig. 7.1 Workflow of HAR and FD with ML, DL, and MH for feature optimized higher accuracy

algorithms actually do navigate through the large search space of possible feature combinations to find feature subsets that will lead to enhanced accuracy resulting into lower computational cost and improved generalization in human activity recognition and fall detection systems. General steps of HAR and FD using machine learning and deep learning models clubbed with metaheuristics optimization techniques ensuring feature optimization and accuracy enhancement.

Feature optimization is a very significant process that needs to be applied for multimodal complex large size HAR datasets having a huge number of features. MH algorithms actually do navigate through the large search space of possible feature combinations to find feature subsets that will lead to enhanced accuracy resulting into lower computational cost and improved generalization in human activity recognition and fall detection systems.

General steps of HAR and FD using machine learning and deep learning models clubbed with metaheuristic optimization techniques ensuring feature optimization and accuracy enhancement are described in Fig. 7.2 for better visualization and understanding.

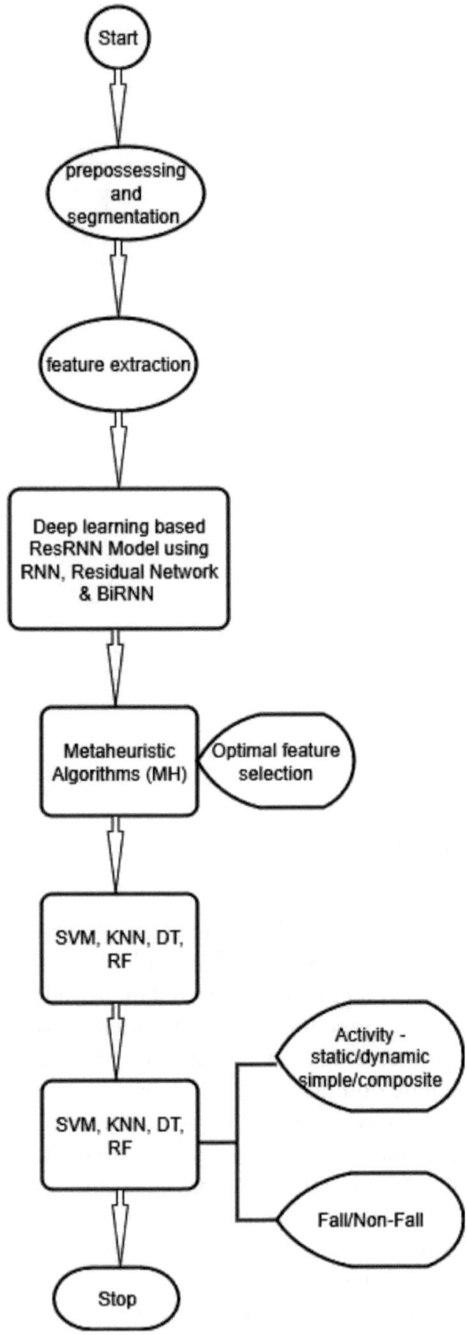

Fig. 7.2 Metaheuristic algorithms applied for feature selection optimization

7.2 Datasets Used in HAR

Human activity recognition (HAR) relies heavily on the quality and structure of datasets used for training and evaluation. However, several challenges are associated with existing HAR datasets, which can impact the performance and generalizability of machine learning models. Below are the key issues:

7.2.1 Key Issues in HAR Datasets

There are a huge number of datasets available for human activity recognition and fall detection, but almost all of them have limitations in terms some of the points as described below. Hence, hybrid datasets are getting popular in which multiple datasets are combined to make it more suitable for performance enhanced HAR.

7.2.1.1 Diverse Activities not Present in All Datasets Available

There are various HAR and FD datasets available, and a number of good research works have already been done in state-of-the-art literatures. But one lack is straightaway identifiable among the datasets and that is availability of diversified activities. Some of the datasets consider very basic activities such as walking, sitting, lying, and running. Whereas some contain complex, composite, concurrent activities like cooking, cleaning utensils, cleaning clothes, doing ironing, operating washing machine, mopping, dining at restaurant, sipping drinks from glass or using straw, etc.

7.2.1.2 Demographic Information is Widely Varied Among the Datasets

- Datasets contain data collected from subject with heterogeneous demographic information regarding age, sex, region, occupation, etc.
- Daily activity monitoring data or health monitoring data collected from one socioeconomic country or region may not be directly applicable to the other space or region.
- Models trained on one set data with limited demography may not often be successful while tested on generalized scenarios across the world.

7.2.1.3 Sensor Placement Inconsistencies

Inertial sensors are smartphone-based or wearable in the form of smart watches, smart bands, etc. If anything extra a subject needs to wear every time at fixed position on his or her body, then these stringent requirements may not be very popularized or acceptable from the usability point of view.

Accuracy of data and classification are dependent on position of device on or around human body, like sensors should be attached to wrist, knee, waist, chest, etc. From this point of view of usability, smartphone-based HAR and FD have got immense acceptance and popularity among the users and the researchers or the developers.

Related to accuracy of data, there are various factors, one such is position or placement of wearable sensors such as accelerometer, pressure sensor, and ECG sensor, orientation of gyroscope sensor is also a very significant factor toward accuracy.

7.2.1.4 Low Sampling Rates or Resolution

- Sampling rates vary in one dataset to another dataset. Some uses low sampling rate, and some uses high or moderately high sampling rate. If the dataset contains data of faster movement of the human body, then the model may not be able to capture data accurately with low sampling rate.
- Data is being captured using heterogeneous sensor devices, all of them are not from same make or manufacturers, not having same or similar resources, and hence, standardization on quality assurance may also not be equal. These inequalities may cause recording of inaccurate data or data may be missed to get recorded leading to missing data. These may lead to noisy feature extraction.

7.2.1.5 Imbalanced Datasets

- In many of the available benchmark datasets, few activities are very common such as sitting, standing, walking, and running irrespective of demography.
- Some of the dynamic activities may not be present or not with sufficient training samples such as jogging, stairs up, stairs down, running, and squatting.
- Lifestyle-related activities and household daily chores like cooking, cleaning, mopping, ironing clothes, etc., also may not be available in many of the datasets.
- Hence, common activities are over-represented and rare, and complex, composite activities are under-represented leading to bias in training.
- Such datasets with uneven distribution of classes with varying samples may lead to wrongful identification of minority classes compared to classes with sufficient samples.

7.2.1.6 Environmental Constraints

May be always the data collection environment and the scenario in which data gathering is done not be the same as that of actual environment in which the HAR and FD system will work in real time. This deviation may lower the accuracy in recognition of the specific activity, fall event.

Several other issues that may lead to less accuracy in HAR and FD could be lack of standardization, privacy, security, labeling ambiguity, etc.

7.3 Datasets Used in Human Activity Recognition (HAR): Description and Comparative Analysis

Human activity recognition (HAR) has emerged as a vital research area due to its applications in health care, smart homes, surveillance, and fitness monitoring. The performance of HAR systems largely depends on the quality and diversity of the datasets used for training and testing. Several benchmark datasets have been developed over the years, each with its own features, modalities, and challenges. This write-up provides an overview of major HAR datasets and a comparative analysis based on key parameters. A comprehensive comparison among different available benchmark HAR datasets is illustrated in details in Table 7.1.

7.3.1 Fall Datasets

HAR datasets are available in large number and reported in state-of-the-art literatures, well explored for various activities over a wide range from simple activities to dynamic, complex activities, activities of daily living (ADL), fitness regime, household chores, etc., as illustrated in the above table.

Fall event detected assisted with IMU sensors, i.e., accelerometer, gyroscope etc., in the form of wearable devices or smartphones are also getting very effective for quality living, and many research papers have illustrated that. A number of datasets are also available as reported in [4, 6], etc., and a comprehensive summary table is given in Table 7.2 for a holistic view on fall datasets.

Sis-Fall: This dataset is unique from the other datasets from the various aspects, one such is in regard to the activities concerned here are not only human activities due to ADL but also multiple types of fall events or actions.

For data collection, an embedded unit comprising of multiple IMU sensors has been exploited, and these are: A Kinets MKL25Z128VLK4 microcontroller which consists of two accelerometers—MMA8451Q and ADXL345 and one ITG3200 gyroscope.

Types of Human Motion Considered

Type 1: Activities of daily living (ADL) consists of static and dynamic activities. Static activities considered are sitting and standing. Dynamic activities considered

Table 7.1 Datasets in HAR: Comparative Analysis

Sl. No.	Dataset	Description	Sensors	Activities	Participants	Sampling rate	Environment	Strengths	Limitations
1	KU-HAR	New dataset for human action and activities	Gyroscopes and accelerometers of smartphones	Simple activities such as standing, sitting, complex activities such as playing table tennis and performing push-ups	90 users, aged between 18 and 34	100 Hz	Indoor and outdoor	18 samples, 90 users, 1945 raw samples, 20,750 subsamples	Class imbalance issue, single modality focus
2	UCI HAR	Sensor data, collected using a Samsung Galaxy S II, on the waist position	IMU sensors, 3-axis accelerometer and gyroscope	6 basic activities—walking, walking upstairs/ downstairs, sitting, standing, lying	30 volunteers	50 Hz	Controlled indoor environment	Clean, well-structured, widely adopted	Basic activities, indoor environment, single modality issue
3	WISDM dataset	Mobile phones and smartwatches, phone in pocket	Accelerometer and gyroscope	Walking, jogging, upstairs, downstairs, sitting, and standing	Over 30	20 Hz (older version), 50 Hz (newer versions)	Semi-controlled	Realistic mobile usage scenarios	Sensor placement variability, some data sparsity, single modality issue
4	PAMAP2 dataset	High-resolution dataset for physical activity monitoring, including heart rate data	Accelerometer, gyroscope, magnetometer, heart rate sensor (sensor fusion)	18 diverse activities including household tasks and sports	9 individuals	100 Hz	Controlled	Rich multimodal data	Small number of subjects

(continued)

Table 7.1 (continued)

Sl. No.	Dataset	Description	Sensors	Activities	Participants	Sampling rate	Environment	Strengths	Limitations
5	Opportunity dataset	Real-world complex activities with object interactions, locomotion and gesture recognition also included	Inertial sensors on body, objects, ambient sensors (sensor fusion)	Locomotion (walking, standing), gestures (open door, drink)	4 subjects	30–100 Hz (varies)	Smart home setting	Multi-sensor, context-aware	High complexity, less number of subjects
6	mHealth dataset	Multiple sensors placement: chest, right wrist, left ankle	Accelerometer, gyroscope, ECG (sensor fusion)	12 activities including jogging, cycling, and standing	10 subjects	50 Hz	Semi-controlled	Multiple body sensor placements, ECG integration	Moderate data size

Table 7.2 HAR and fall datasets

Sl. No.	Dataset	Data points	Time window (s)	Sensors used	Filter used/segmentation
1	KU-HAR	300	3	Accelerometer	Low-pass filter to remove noise
2	OPPORTUNITY	64	2.133	IMU sensors	For the segmentation at a rate of 50%, overlapping have been employed
3	PAMAP2	54 columns of sensor reading	5	IMU sensors, heart rate sensor	Butterworth filter
4	WISDM	Cut-off frequency 10 Hz	128	Accelerometer, gyroscope	Butterworth low-pass filter, overlapping with 50%
5	UCI-HAR	50 Hz	2.56	Accelerometer	Overlapping with 50%
6	UniMiBSHAR	150	3	Smartphone accelerometer	Segmentation done
7	Sis-Fall	600	3	Accelerometer, gyroscope	Low-pass filter

are jogging, walking, stairs up and down, jumping, and stumbling while walking, etc.

Type 2: Fall events—Fall may occur during human movement. The movement could be during movements done for daily living. Based on different activity or movement or motion from which fall may occur, 15 different types of fall actions have been considered.

Fall Actions Considered

Fall forward, fall backward, fall while jogging, fall while getting up, fall while sitting down, etc.

Subjects contributing data: Total human activity and fall data have been collected from a total number of 36 people, among them 15 elderly users with 8 male and 7 female. 23 were young people, and among them 12 were female and 11 male. 600 data points have been used, and the time window used was 3 s. At data preprocessing stage, a low-pass filter has been used to remove noise.

Data cleaning, filtration, and segmentation used in datasets are already discussed in the previous chapters of this book, and the readers may please refer to the previous content.

7.4 Case Studies and Scenario Based on HAR Systems

7.4.1 Channel Status Information (CSI)-Based HAR

Mekruksavanich et al. [7] used an unique approach based on a deep learning network and the type of the data. RSSI, i.e., received signal strength indicator is popularly used in various applications but instead of that potential offered by WiFi-based detection techniques, the authors have utilized channel status information (CSI). The authors proposed a hybrid deep learning network called CNN-GRU-AttNet that exploits CNN and GRU to extract informative spatio-temporal features from raw CSI data automatically efficient tasks classification. To further improve recognition accuracy, an attention mechanism has been integrated into the network that prioritizes important features and time steps.

The network consists of five layers:

- The input layer
- Two CNN layers
- A GRU layer
- An attention layer
- A fully connected layer and
- an output layer.

For performance evaluation of the proposed models, they have used two public datasets: CSI-HAR and Stan WIFI. The activities considered are the dynamic activities we often perform due to fitness regime or daily cores. The activities considered are: walking, running, sitting, lying down, standing up, bending, and falling. For experimental results and performance evaluation purpose, fivefold cross-validation technique is used. Comparative performance analysis is done implementing different deep learning models such as: CNN, LSTM, BiLSTM, GRU, and BiGRU. The results show exceptional efficacy in the classification of HAR activities, superior to the five basic DL models, producing an average accuracy of 99.62%, an accuracy of 99.61%, and an $F1$ score of 99.61% in all movements.

7.4.2 Smartphone-Based HAR

Smartphone has IMU sensors such as accelerometer, gyroscope, etc., that sense movement of human being and detect activities performed due to activities of daily living. Activities could be static as well as dynamic and can be due to fitness regime, due to daily chores in household activities, etc. The raw signals are analyzed using machine learning models for feature extraction and activity class identification. Multimodal sensors and data are utilized in smartphone-based HAR. Smartphone camera sensor can be used to capture videos or images of a person's activity, and applying deep learning models, activities could be recognized. Sensors fusion, information fusion, data fusion, etc., are utilized for accuracy enhancement. Several public datasets such as UCI HAR public dataset and WISDM dataset have been used in different literatures.

The sensor data from the triaxial accelerometer and gyroscope used in this study came from the "WISDM Activity and Biometrics for Smartphones and Smartwatches" published by Weiss [8].

7.4.3 RADAR-Based Fall Detection (FD) System

Scenario description: In a smart home setting, a RADAR-based HAR prototype is installed in the living room. It monitors an elderly individual. If the system detects a fall (sharp vertical movement with specific micro-Doppler signature), it instantly triggers an emergency alert to caregivers. Unlike vision-based systems, the RADAR respects privacy while functioning in darkness or through walls [9].

7.4.4 Prototype Components

A RADAR-based HAR system prototype typically consists of the following components: **RADAR Sensor**: Frequency-modulated continuous wave (FMCW) or mmWave RADAR (e.g., Texas Instruments IWR6843) operating in 60 GHz or 77 GHz bands. This system consists of following major components:

Processing Unit: Comprises a real-time embedded processor (e.g., TI DCA1000EVM or Raspberry Pi) that collects and processes sensor data.

Signal Processing Pipeline: Includes (i) Range–Doppler map generation, (ii) Micro-Doppler signature extraction, and (iii) Spectrogram or feature matrix creation.

To process and analyze, a number of machine learning algorithms have been used: CNNs, RNNs, or SVMs.

These algorithms have been trained to classify several human activities such as walking, sitting, falling down, or waving based on the Doppler signatures.

Now if readers are eager to know basic working principles of such RADAR-based activity and movement recognition systems, then this brief illustration may help.

Unlike sensor-based traditional HAR and FD systems, the subject is here free to move in the specified region without being concerned about the data collecting device to be attached to body in specific positions or orientation. Here, the RADAR transmits continuous RF signals into the surrounding environment. Human motion causes Doppler shifts in the reflected signals due to body part movements. These micro-Doppler signatures are extracted and analyzed to distinguish between various human activities. The extracted features are then classified by a machine learning model trained on labeled motion data.

This allows the system to recognize activities without relying on cameras, ensuring both privacy and usability in environments like elder care, smart homes, and hospitals [10].

7.4.5 Sensor Fusion-Based HAR

When heterogeneous data is collected using different types of sensors and the integrated for application in human activity recognition (HAR) and fall detection (FD), then the systems are called sensor fusion-based HAR and FD. Heterogeneous sensors combined in such systems are mainly IMU sensors such as accelerometers, gyroscopes, magnetometers, may be few a times barometers or camera sensors, clubbed with acoustic sensors, pressure sensors, etc. Fusion-based approaches are basically preferred over single-type sensor-based systems because system's performance in terms of accuracy, reliability for human activity recognition, and fall detection got enhanced. The limitations of individual sensors can be overcome by combining data from multiple sources, and also, robustness in real-world environments gets enhanced.

7.5 Scenario-Based Study

In [11], the authors experimented with a model for orientation-independent HAR with five classes using deep neural network (DNN). Activities considered are mainly for patients: (i) Slow and assisted walking, (ii) Using wheelchair, etc. The specific features of this model are as follows:

- It is orientation-agnostic, data augmentation technique is applied.
- GENActiv wearable device embedded with high-resolution triaxial accelerometer sensor is attached on trunk of a person for acceleration measurement
- Six activities considered—lying in bed, upright posture, walking, wheelchair transport, stair ascent, and stair descent
- Data collection was done from 20 subjects: 10 male, 10 female, age range 18–65 years, in a simulated hospital environment.

Total 23,000 labeled segments have been collected, for training purpose, 50% of collected data have been used, and for testing 25% and for validation 25%, data has been utilized. Fixed-length sliding window technique, with 6 s length and overlap of 50%, has been used for data segmentation purpose. From each acceleration segment, total 86 numbers of time domain and frequency domain features have been extracted. DNN and SVM have been used, and accuracies achieved are 94.5% and 83.35%.

7.6 Reference Sensor Attached to the Environment-Based Human Activity and Movement Recognition

Velasco et al. [12] used the HAR approach to understand human behavior by analyzing data representative of domestic routines. This work targets to study relation between ADL along with place and time of occurrences.

The research outcomes are beneficial from different perspectives:

- This information is helpful for healthcare professionals to assess the health status of patients
- Family members can keep track of the habits of near ones
- Architects can design home giving priority to the accessibility and movement pattern of the residents.

The database used is the knowledge discovery database (KDD) approach with the data analyst variant as a key player in the knowledge discovery process. The KDD approach is an interactive and iterative knowledge discovery process that identifies relationships between data that must be valid, new, potentially useful, and understandable.

The performance evaluation parameters used are as follows:

- The sequence of places visited, times of day at which they are visited, and average duration of visits.
- The signals acquired using PIR sensors connected to a Raspberry Pi4. These are placed in each of the room considered.
- Subjects in concern worn a BLE device that emits RSSI which changed with change in position of the subject. Thus the transitions between positions can be detected with the varied RSSI.
- Performance evaluation has been done including all the stakeholders such as users, architects, and health professionals.

7.6.1 Wearable Sensor-Based HAR

Wearable sensors are arguably the most ubiquitous and natural option for HAR, as they are attached directly to or worn on the subject, offering intimate and continuous body kinematic and physiological state measurements. Their close proximity to the activity source facilitates the collection of fine-grained, high-fidelity data, rendering them essential for numerous HAR applications. Inertial measurement units (IMUs): Inertial measurement units (IMUs) are sensor combinations that are normally composed of accelerometers, gyroscopes, and occasionally magnetometers. They are common in contemporary smartphones, smartwatches, and specialized wearable devices, serving as the core component of a majority of HAR systems because they have the capacity to record detailed motion dynamics.

i. Accelerometers: An accelerometer detects nongravitational acceleration, or proper acceleration, of the device. For HAR, accelerometers usually acquire linear acceleration on three orthogonal axes (X, Y, Z). This information is essential to identify changes in speed, direction, and orientation. From patterns in acceleration, one can even recognize walking, running, jumping, falling, and tiny gestures. For example, rhythmic oscillations in acceleration data may correspond to walking, whereas abrupt large changes may represent a fall. The naked acceleration signal usually has both gravitational and body motion parts, which are usually separated in preprocessing to exclude the movement-specific acceleration.
ii. Gyroscopes: Gyroscope measures angular velocity or rate of rotation about an axis. Like accelerometers, gyroscopes of HAR systems tend to give information along three orthogonal axes. Whereas accelerometers pick up on linear motion, gyroscopes are required to capture rotational movement, e.g., rotation, torsion, or swinging of limbs. The fusion of accelerometer and gyroscope information offers a more thorough understanding of human movement and better differential diagnosis between actions that may have the same linear acceleration pattern but with different rotations. For instance, running and walking may share similar accelerations, but arm swings and rotations of the body would be clearly recorded by a gyroscope.
iii. Magnetometers: A magnetometer quantifies the direction and magnitude of magnetic fields. Magnetometers are utilized in IMUs to measure absolute orientation against the Earth's north magnetic pole. The data is essential for calibrating the drift that may pile up in the readings of accelerometers and gyroscopes over time, which phenomenon is known as drift. Through supplying a stable reference for the purpose of orientation, magnetometers increase the precision of tracking motion and activity recognition, especially for activities with direction or orientation in space changes. Magnetometers may, however, be sensitive to disturbance by external magnetic fields, a factor that should be taken into consideration at data collection and analysis times.

Human activity recognition (HAR) with machine learning has attracted broad interest because it could be applied in healthcare, home automation, and fitness tracking. As wearable sensors and Internet of things (IoT) devices have become increasingly popular, researchers have proposed several ML-based frameworks for automated activity classification. These methods take input from accelerometers, gyroscopes, and other movement sensors to identify physical activities such as walking, sitting, and standing with great precision. The incorporation of ML methods improves the accuracy, flexibility, and expandability of HAR systems, which is highly appropriate for context-aware and real-time applications. There are various studies conducted regarding IoT and ML integration to recognize human activities. Wearable sensors and intelligent devices facilitate real-time monitoring of people with health issues, especially the elderly. Methods like SVM, random forest, and K-NN have been found to be highly accurate to differentiate activities and facilitate independent living and preventive medical care [13]. Current studies in human activity recognition (HAR) utilize machine learning and deep learning algorithms to recognize activities from inertial sensor data. Methods such as CNNs, RNNs, and hybrid approaches significantly enhance accuracy for recognition. The models provide real-time analysis in IoT applications, which can be used for health care, surveillance, and smart applications [14]. Current research in HAR focuses on applying inertial sensor data with machine learning and deep learning algorithms toward effective activity classification. Methods such as axis-wise feature extraction, CNNs, and ensemble methods have improved recognition performance. These developments form the basis of reliable, real-time HAR systems in healthcare, smart environments, and wearable technology [8]. Current studies on human activity recognition (HAR) involve machine and deep learning models based on inertial and thermal sensor data. Methodologies such as CNNs, SVMs, and axis-based feature extraction have been enhanced to increase recognition accuracy. These advancements enable real-time, unobtrusive monitoring in health care, smart homes, and IoT environments [15]. Human activity recognition (HAR) research employs more and more triaxial accelerometer recordings with machine learning for the identification of sophisticated behaviors such as coughing in motion. Methods such as FFT feature extraction, SVM, and decision trees proved useful in activity discrimination, which expands applications in mobile health monitoring and unobtrusive behavior sensing [16]. Recent HAR studies employ micro-Doppler radar and machine learning to identify faint human movements. Time–frequency representation features allow precise walking, running, and falling classification. Noncontact sensing techniques augment infrared and inertial methods, enhancing HAR applications in health care, surveillance, and ambient intelligence [17]. Recent HAR research contrasts deep learning and conventional models such as SVM in sports movement classification, for instance, table tennis strokes. Results indicate that CNNs perform better than SVMs in extracting motion details from sensor data. Such observations underscore the increasing power of deep models for fine-grained activity recognition and sport performance analysis [18]. Human activity recognition works more and more often uses wearable sensors and machine learning for rehabilitation. Experiments categorize shoulder exercises by employing algorithms such as SVM, k-NN, and random forest with high accuracy. These techniques provide computer-aided feedback in physiotherapy, improving patient surveillance, quality of rehabilitation, and minimizing the necessity for continuous clinical oversight [19]. Machine learning methods are applied more and more for real-time gesture recognition from continuous wave radar signals. Features extracted from the Doppler spectrograms enable SVM and k-NN classifiers to detect at high accuracy. Contactless radar-based systems improve human activity recognition, especially in scenarios where wearable sensors become impractical [20]. Recent research in affective computing investigates emotion detection with multichannel EEG signals and machine learning. Robust frameworks employ signal preprocessing, feature extraction, and classifiers such as SVM and ANN to provide good classification of emotions. These systems complement human activity recognition systems and provide better insights into cognitive and emotional human states [21]. In [22], Huang et al. proposed a new multiscale hierarchical adaptive network structure for HAR called HMA Conv-LSTM. To validate the efficacy of the proposed model, the authors carried out experiments on several public HAR datasets: Opportunity, PAMAP2, USC-HAD, and Skoda.

7.6.2 Fall Detection Scenarios

Sensor-based fall detection strategies are many, following is a representative diagram, Fig. 7.3. Among all these methods of fall detection that actually varies mainly based on the type of data and sensors are being used in each method. Among these, smartphone-based fall detection methods are getting increased popularity both ways, among the users as well as researchers (Figs. 7.4 and 7.5 and Table 7.3).

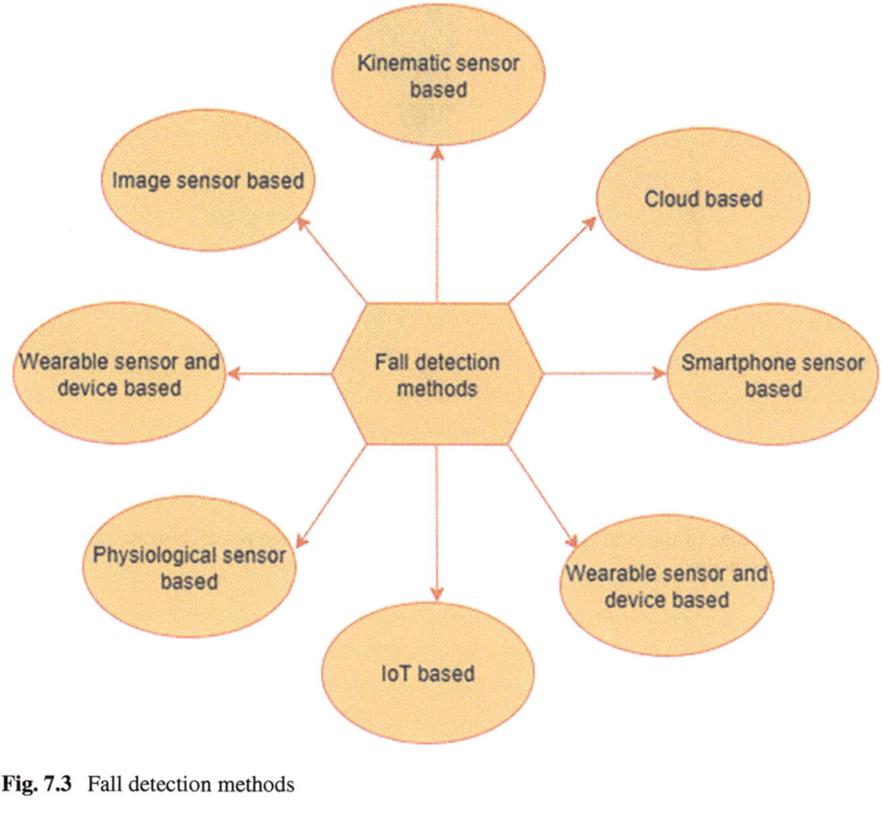

Fig. 7.3 Fall detection methods

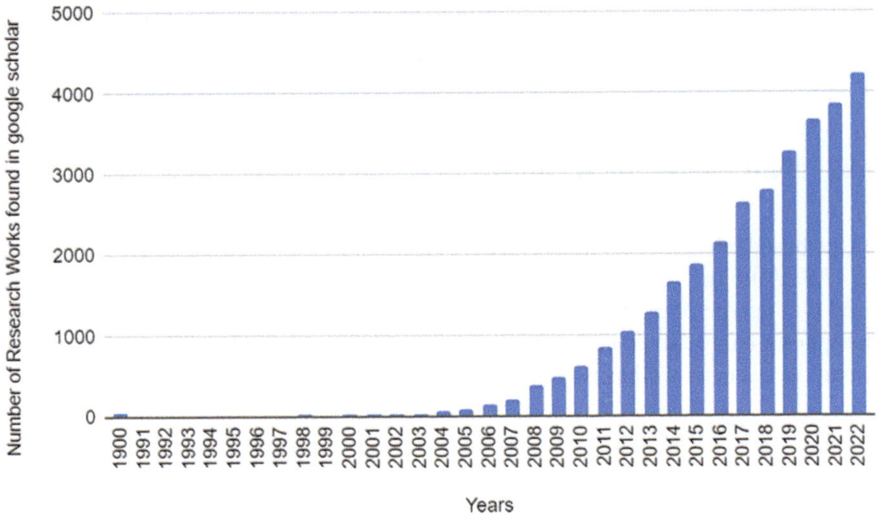

Fig. 7.4 Fall detection research papers found in Google Scholar from 1990 to 2022

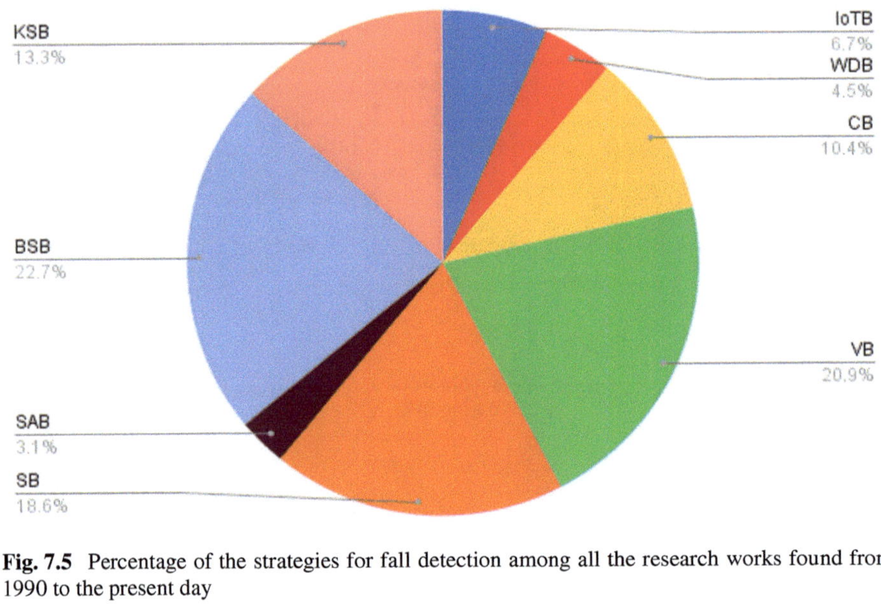

Fig. 7.5 Percentage of the strategies for fall detection among all the research works found from 1990 to the present day

Table 7.3 Percentage of different methods of HAR

Methods	IoT-based (IoTB)	Wearable device-based (WDB)	Cloud-based (CB)	Vision-based (VB)	Smartphone-based (SB)	Sound analysis-based (SAB)	Biomedical signal-based (BSB)	Kinematic signal-based (KSB)
Percentage	6.682692308%	4.480769231%	10.38461538%	20.86538462%	18.55769231%	3.067307692%	22.69230769%	13.26923077%

7.7 Conclusion

Each HAR dataset offers unique benefits and is suited to different types of research. The UCI HAR dataset remains a standard benchmark due to its simplicity, while PAMAP2 and Opportunity provide rich, complex data ideal for advanced models. However, challenges such as limited participant diversity, unrealistic environments, and inconsistent sensor placement still persist. Future research should aim to develop more diverse, scalable, and real-world applicable HAR datasets to build robust models.

References

1. Wazwaz, A. A., Amin, K. M., Semari, N. A., & Ghanem, T. F. (2023). Enhancing human activity recognition using features reduction in IoT edge and Azure cloud. *Decision Analytics Journal, 8*, Article 100282.
2. Saeed, U., Shah, S. Y., Shah, S. A., Ahmad, J., Alotaibi, A. A., Althobaiti, T., Ramzan, N., Alomainy, A., & Abbasi, Q. H. (2021). Discrete human activity recognition and fall detection by combining FMCW RADAR data of heterogeneous environments for independent assistive living. *Electronics, 10*(18), 2237.
3. Khasnobish, A., Ray, A., Chowdhury, A., Rani, S., Chakravarty, T., & Pal, A. (2021, June). Novel composite motion extraction from velocity signature of FMCW radar for activity recognition. In *2021 21st International Radar Symposium (IRS)* (pp. 1–8). IEEE.
4. The applications of meteheuristics for human activity recognition and fall detection using wearable sensors: A comprehensive analysis. https://www.kaggle.com/datasets/uttejkumarkandagatla/fall-detection-dataset
5. Al-Qaness, M. A., Helmi, A. M., Dahou, A., & Elaziz, M. A. (2022). The applications of metaheuristics for human activity recognition and fall detection using wearable sensors: A comprehensive analysis. *Biosensors, 12*(10), 821.
6. Mekruksavanich, S., Phaphan, W., Hnoohom, N., & Jitpattanakul, A. (2023). Attention-based hybrid deep learning network for human activity recognition using WiFi channel state information. *Applied Sciences, 13*(15), 8884.
7. Kim, C., & Lee, W. (2023). Human activity recognition by the image type encoding method of 3-axial sensor data. *Applied Sciences, 13*(8), 4961.
8. *People counting and activity recognition using mmWave radar sensors.* Application Report, Texas Instruments. (2019). https://www.ti.com/lit/pdf/spracv1
9. Adib, F., Mao, H., Kabelac, Z., Katabi, D., & Miller, R. C. (2015). Smart homes that monitor breathing and heart rate. In *Proceedings of the 33rd Annual ACM Conference on Human Factors in Computing Systems (CHI '15)* (pp. 837–846). https://doi.org/10.1145/2702123.2702200
10. Newaz, N. T., & Hanada, E. (2023). The methods of fall detection: A literature review. *Sensors, 23*(11), 5212.
11. Arribas Velasco, A., McGrory, J., & Berry, D. (2023). An evaluation study on the analysis of people's domestic routines based on spatial, temporal and sequential aspects. *Applied Sciences, 13*(19), 10608.
12. Mittal, P. (2022). Machine learning (ML) based human activity recognition model using smart sensors in IoT environment. In *2022 12th International Conference on Cloud Computing, Data Science & Engineering (Confluence)*. IEEE.
13. Mehmood, K., Ali Imran, H., & Latif, U. (2020). Hardensenet: A 1d densenet inspired convolutional neural network for human activity recognition with inertial sensors. In *2020 IEEE 23rd International Multitopic Conference (INMIC)*. IEEE.

14. Mishra, R., et al. (2024). Optimizing activity recognition through dominant axis identification in inertial sensors. *IEEE Sensors Letters*.
15. Rezaei, A., et al. (2022). An unobtrusive human activity recognition system using low resolution thermal sensors, machine and deep learning. *IEEE Transactions on Biomedical Engineering, 70*(1), 115–124.
16. FFT spectrum spread with machine learning (ML) analysis of triaxial acceleration from shirt pocket and torso for sensing coughs while walking.
17. Wang, Z., et al. (2023). Recognition of approximate motions of human based on micro-Doppler features. *IEEE Sensors Journal, 23*(11), 12388–12397.
18. Sassi, M., et al. (2024). Classification of shoulder rehabilitation exercises by using wearable systems and machine learning algorithms. *IEEE Sensors Journal, 24*(14), 22934–22944.
19. Tabrizi, S. S., Pashazadeh, S., & Javani, V. (2020). Comparative study of table tennis forehand strokes classification using deep learning and SVM. *IEEE Sensors Journal, 20*(22), 13552–13561.
20. Ehrnsperger, M. G., et al. (2020). Real-time gesture detection based on machine learning classification of continuous wave radar signals. *IEEE Sensors Journal, 21*(6), 8310–8322.
21. Nalwaya, A., Das, K., & Pachori, R. B. (2024). An automated framework for human emotion detection from multichannel EEG signals. *IEEE Sensors Journal, 24*(13), 20920–20927.
22. Huang, Q., Xie, W., Li, C., Wang, Y., & Liu, Y. (2023). Human action recognition based on hierarchical multi-scale adaptive conv-long short-term memory network. *Applied Sciences, 13*(19), 10560.
23. Weiss, G. M. (2019). WISDM smartphone and smartwatch activity and biometrics dataset. *UCI Machine Learning Repository: WISDM Smartphone and Smartwatch Activity and Biometrics Dataset Data Set, 7*(133190–133202), 5.
24. Bibbo, L., & Vellasco, M. M. (2023). Human activity recognition (HAR) in healthcare. *Applied Sciences, 13*(24), 13009.
25. Fridriksdottir, E., & Bonomi, A. G. (2020). Accelerometer-based human activity recognition for patient monitoring using a deep neural network. *Sensors, 20*(22), 6424.

Chapter 8
Conclusion

This chapter is the final chapter that will summarize all the contributions and unique features of this book to the reader with highlight of future scope. This chapter put summarizing eye on the important and significant content of each chapter illustrated before with all minute details, information, and description, illustrations to read thoroughly by the interested readers, and at the end the reader will get the footprint of all the chapters in a nutshell for getting the holistic view.

The book is organized with the planned and well-structured framework comprising of total 8 chapters including introduction and conclusion. Chapters 2–7 illustrate all theoretical, fundamental, and technical details of different concepts on data, algorithms, models, methods, tools, techniques, etc. This book is a handbook or a guide to the beginners in the well-explored and future-promising, high-demanding applications developed with human activity recognition (HAR) and fall detection (FD) for benefit of the human living. We, the human being do movements naturally during our daily living for many purposes: just to move at indoor or at outdoor we walk, run, do stairs up or do stairs down, etc. We may be in sitting, standing, or laying postures, and these are static activities. For fitness regime, people may do running, walking, jogging, jumping, squatting, do sit-ups, push-ups, etc., and these are dynamic activities. During household daily chores, people do several complex activities such as cooking, washing clothes with hand or using washing machine, pressing clothes with iron, mopping, etc. Also some activities could be concurrent such as walking while brushing teeth, walking while eating, dancing, and listening to music, eating while watching TV, etc. Elderly people are only comfortable with static activities, and they are prone to fall very often. Diseased people are convenient with slower activities such as slow walking, sitting, moving by wheelchair, walking using walking stick, etc. Both the elderly or diseased elderly are prone to fall due to foot imbalance, body imbalance, stumble due to obstacle while walking, etc. So the system should be able to recognize activities as well as fall to generate alert and extend timely support. Now the big question that comes to the brilliant minds is how these could be remotely done maintaining accuracy, security privacy, reliability, robustness, etc. The

S. Biswas, *Machine Learning and Deep Learning in Human Activity Recognition and Fall Detection*, Signals and Communication Technology,
https://doi.org/10.1007/978-3-032-09241-0_8

answer is technology. Now, what technologies we are talking about? The technologies that have been developed in much advanced form are sensors, Internet of things, cloud computing, VLSI, 5G communications, machine learning, camera sensor, deep learning, artificial intelligence, etc.

So, when a people actually does some activity, may be running or walking or jumping, we with our bare eyes can see their body or body parts movement and recognize the label of the activity from our previous learning. May be the person is jumping at roof and I am not seeing his movements but I can listen to the sound pattern, intensity, frequency, etc., and can identify the movement or type of movement again from our learning by experience. Now, when the person is at remote end and I am unable to see or hear him/her, then how his current posture or activity could be correctly identified? Here the sensors do the tasks of ears and eyes. The basic, primitive, easy to use, efficient, low cost, usable sensors used in HAR and FD are: Accelerometer and gyroscope may be available embedded in wearable devices or in smartphones, the indispensable object of human life nowadays. Basically what these sensors do? Accelerometer senses body acceleration due to specific movement and extracting features of the movement, finds the movement pattern, and recognizes specific activities like sitting, standing, walking, lying etc. Gyroscope plays pivotal role along with accelerometer when direction or orientation is important like stairs up or stair down, walking toward right or left etc.

The book begins with the introduction chapter that describes essential fundamental concepts on human activity recognition, fall monitoring and detection, application of HAR and FD in health monitoring and cares, in geriatric care, i.e., health care of diseased elderly, different framework of HAR-based health care, discussion, and insight on sustainability of such systems through rigorous performance evaluation, etc. Basic concepts on sensors, IoT, cloud, AI and ML and their roles in HAR and FD systems have been well demonstrated. Initial conceptualization of data collection, data processing, features, training, testing, validation, activity recognition etc., general framework of IoT based HAR system and it's working principle etc. are also described for everyone's understanding. Different types of heterogeneous sensors used for various data collection linked with human activity such as acceleration data, movement direction or orientation data, physiological parameters like heart rate, pulse rate, body temperature, breathing rate, foot pressure, etc. Surroundings sound could help to find the place of the person doing certain activity, for that acoustic sensor can be used, and use of camera sensor, drone, or satellite images, RADAR technology, etc., are also being used for HAR and FD. Some basic preliminaries on methodologies or intelligent models based on artificial intelligence, machine learning, deep learning, reinforcement learning, etc., are also touched upon.

Concepts on use of sensors and positions of sensors on human body to acquire vital signals along with use of smartphone sensors with self-illustrative diagrams are also helpful to clear with the introductory basic concepts.

Chapter 2 moves on to illustrating fundamental concepts, introduction and overview of enabling smart technologies—sensors, Internet of things, machine learning, deep learning, cloud, etc., that help to design, develop, and implement the system starting from raw data collection to processing to pattern recognition to knowledge generation, appropriate alert, or feedback to the concerned authorities for timely action specifically in time-critical scenarios like health care, etc.

This chapter gives the reader and the researchers a complete guided tour through the different enabling technologies of HAR systems and brief discussion on the enabling technologies, their fundamental working principles, their specific roles in HAR, what exact functions they perform at which stage or phase of HAR, etc. Sensors ranging from wearable to smartphone embedded to physiological to environmental, etc., Internet of things and its role in HAR, cloud computing and its specific roles being performed, machine learning algorithms that do data processing for learning and identification, etc., are well elaborated. These introductory, basic concepts actually build the basics upon which the real-time HAR application would be developed with ensured good performance.

Chapter 3 is elaborated on machine learning in human activity recognition using smartphone sensors, fundamental concepts of machine learning, smartphone as sensor hub, accelerometer sensor, gyroscope sensor, machine learning models in HAR, application of accelerometer and gyroscope sensor data in HAR, dataset analysis for better insight, etc. This chapter addresses the growing need for effective, nonintrusive health monitoring for human being and in specific cases for elderly individuals, particularly those living alone with chronic conditions. It proposes a novel system that utilizes the built-in sensors of ubiquitous smart devices like smartphones and smart watches such as accelerometers and gyroscopes—to monitor physical activity and vital signs without requiring additional wearable devices. HAR-based systems could further be utilized for healthcare systems in different needs such as health monitoring, disease monitoring, disease detection, and prediction. Body vitals sensed by physiological sensors such as heart rate and pulse rate during different activities would be transmitted to a processing server for analysis and knowledge extraction of normal or abnormal parameter values in case of any specific high intense dynamic activity, and accordingly, alert could be generated for early detection of health issues and timely intervention by appropriate authority. The study also highlights a critical gap in existing research, where most systems fail to integrate activity recognition with vital sign monitoring and often overlook transitional movements between activities. In such cases, sensor fusion approach combines data from multiple types of sensors or devices such as IMU sensors of smartphones, smart watches, wearable physiological sensors such as pulse oximeter sensor, and blood pressure sensors—to track both health parameters and a broad range of ADL, i.e., activities of daily living. Advanced algorithms are used to analyze these large data and categorize users based on their fitness level, enabling personalized healthcare management. This chapter enlists and describes working of advanced machine learning algorithms for recognizing activities from raw sensory data. This comprehensive solution offers a promising direction for activity recognition, fall detection, proactive health monitoring, elderly care, etc.

Different existing human activity recognition systems as described by the researchers in various literatures present in front of the eager learners about set of activities considered such as walking, running, sitting, standing, walking upstairs, walking downstairs, biking, cycling, sitting on chair, and sitting on floor. Machine learning algorithms popularly and successfully used are Naïve Bayes, (NB), decision tree, support vector machines (SVM), KNN, multilayer perceptron (MLP), Naïve Bayes, random forest, etc. These machine learning models efficiently work on sensory data. Nowadays, there are several image and video capturing devices being installed at home, offices, airports, big shopping malls, at outdoors in different strategic positions by the government or administrative authorities like busy traffic signals in metro cities, on highways, expressways, etc. Also drone surveillance is being used at increasing rate at both urban and rural areas, and these drone captured videos or images are also the data source for human activity recognition or fall detection. Several applications are being developed where sensors are used to get the data on the environment in which the person is performing the activity. For that acoustic sensors are used to capture background noises along with RADAR signals or satellite images also being used for HAR and FD. Hence, data types are varied and can be text, numeric values, image, video, audio signals, etc. In machine learning, feature extraction is manual or handcrafted, and for large, complex dataset with high dimensionality, manual feature extraction is a trivial job. Deep learning gets immense popularity in processing image video and complex signals as it has automated features extraction property, and this made this paradigm much popular in case of large, complex image, video, audio, complex signals individually or as a fusion dataset through data fusion, information fusion, and features fusion techniques. CNN, LSTM, ANN, DNN, and RNN as individual deep learning models or as a combination of multiple algorithms such as CNN-LSTM, deep CNN (DCNN), ANN-LSTM, and deep recurrent neural network (DRNN) work efficiently on image, video data-based HAR and FD and given improved accuracy over machine learning algorithms such as SVM and KNN.

Human activity recognition (HAR) is an area which has gained increasing importance in health care like the rise of wearable sensors and mobile health technologies. With the method of being capturing and analyzing patterns in human motion, HAR systems are used to offer a noninvasive method to monitor daily activities and can detect irregularities that may signal the onset or progression of disease. Chapter 4 is structured to present the power and efficiency of deep learning models in HAR. When attached with deep learning techniques, HAR becomes a most powerful tool that can enhance the accuracy and efficiency of disease identification across a wide range of medical conditions. Deep learning models, such as convolutional neural networks (CNNs), recurrent neural networks (RNNs), and long short-term memory (LSTM) networks, have shown an exceptionally good performance in interpreting time-series data from sensors like accelerometers and gyroscopes. Such models can learn continuous patterns automatically from the given/collected raw data without needing extensive manual feature engineering. This capability makes them allow to detect notable deviations in movement and behavior that might get unnoticed in traditional clinical assessments. Many applications of deep learning-enabled HAR in disease detection are diverse in nature. For neurodegenerative diseases like Parkinson's or Alzheimer's, these specific models help identify early signs of motor and cognitive decline by analyzing walking patterns, tremors, or daily activity levels. In patients healing stage from strokes, HAR systems help in several areas like monitoring mobility improvements and tailoring rehabilitation plans. In the same way, in chronic conditions such as in diabetes or cardiovascular disease, it changes in physical activity which are detected through HAR might be serve as early warnings or early indicators of health degradation. The incorporation of HAR and deep learning can transform disease management by enabling real-time and continuous health monitoring outside of clinical setups. This is the kind of shift which supports earlier detection, personalized treatment, and proactive interventions in several ways, which are critical in many areas like in managing long-term health conditions. Moreover, this unique and unobtrusive nature of sensor-based monitoring surely encourages consistent data collection to make it easier for clinicians to gain insights into patient health over time. This chapter can highlight this transformative role of deep learning in advancing HAR applications in disease identification by suggesting a promising future for intelligent, data-driven healthcare solutions.

Chapter 5 completely covers the fall detection systems using machine learning and deep learning algorithms. The rapid evolution of wearable sensors and mobile edge computing has heralded a new era in health and safety monitoring, enabling continuous, unobtrusive surveillance of human motion for at-risk populations. Human activity recognition (HAR) systems classify routine behaviors—such as walking, sitting, standing, and lying down—by interpreting streams of accelerometer and gyroscope data. Fall detection (FD), a critical subset of HAR, focuses on identifying abrupt, potentially injurious events that disproportionately affect elderly individuals and patients with movement disorders. Traditional FD methods typically apply simple threshold rules to the signal vector magnitude (SVM) of triaxial acceleration, triggering alarms whenever SVM exceeds preset limits. However, such rule-based solutions often misinterpret fast sit-to-stand motions, stumbles, or device knocks as genuine falls, resulting in high false alarm rates and caregiver "alarm fatigue." In response, modern approaches integrate machine learning (ML) to extract rich time–frequency features and learn complex decision boundaries that more accurately discriminate between routine movements and dangerous falls, improving both sensitivity and specificity in real-world deployments.

Chapter 6 is framed with a plan to focus on the issues associate with single sensor-based HAR and fall detection. The use of a single sensor in the HAR task has been unreliable because most sensors have limited information due to sensor deprivation, limited spatial coverage, occlusion, imprecision, and uncertainty.

In order to address the issues of using one sensor and improve the performance (measured mainly by accuracy, recall, sensitivity, and specificity, etc., described earlier) of the recognition, researchers have proposed methods of multi-sensor data fusion. Using multiple sensors for recognizing human activities makes sense because the information missed by one sensor can sometimes be provided by the others and also the imprecision of a single sensor can often be compensated by other similar ones. Many works have shown an accuracy improvement compared to single sensor. Now, there is a wide variety of methods for combining the information acquired from several similar or different sensors, and there are active research areas called "sensor fusion", "information fusion", and similar ones, which have dedicated journals, conferences, and so forth. Even when restricting our attention to multi-sensor fusion in the context of HAR, there are hundreds of specific works having used many variants of combinations of fusion methods, and each author claims to have achieved better results than others, so the need for putting some order in this area seems evident.

Chapter 7 is aimed to illustrate the design, development, and deployment strategies keeping an eye on the challenges that the current systems, methodologies, tools, and technologies may impose while implementing in real time. The challenges are at different stages of human activity recognition and fall detection systems and also are at different levels as well.

First of all, any design, development, and deployment begins with data collection or capturing or gathering, and here, the data capturing elements are mainly sensors. Now if we look at evolution history of HAR, the sensors used for raw data collection were primarily IMU sensors in wearable form, i.e., accelerometer or gyroscope. And also another type of input data collection devices used primarily has been camera sensors and then CCTV cameras installed in strategic positions at indoor or at outdoor, thus enabling HAR and FD at both the places without any movement area restrictions. Also in this later system, the user or the subject need not to be bothered about his or her involvement in data collection or generation, rather he or she in free to move, and knowingly or unknowingly the person is contributing in data gathering.

Also, initial methods or systems have been designed and developed to handle with homogeneous type of sensors gathering homogeneous data and that could be either text, image, numeric values, videos, etc. Applying threshold-based approach or applying supervised machine learning algorithms such as SVM, DT, NB, and KNN on single modal data, accuracy of HAR and FD systems in real time was not giving very good level of accuracy.

With the development of embedded technologies, availability of tiny, lightweight, affordable different types of sensors such as physiological sensors, pressure sensor, environmental sensors, piezoelectric sensors, and acoustic sensors, and combining inertial sensors with one or more of other sensory data, the practical systems being developed nowadays as are utilizing multimodal data. Hence, data size, data complexity, and volume all are increasing. To handle with such huge dataset, single, base machine learning-based classifiers such as SVM and KNN are not sufficient to give higher accuracy.

Future Scope

This book is a very good reference to all interested beginners or active researchers of the domain of human activity recognition and fall detection systems for several purposes as follows:

- Monitoring of activities of daily living (ADL)
- Detection of fall events
- HAR application in health care—for disease detection, disease prediction, etc.
- Prediction of fall events in disease elderly

- Activity monitoring for surveillance to detect any suspicious human body or body part movement.
- Human activity monitoring of daily household chores
- Human activity monitoring of daily fitness regime of a person
- Human activity monitoring for rehabilitation of diseased elderly
- Fall detection module exploiting smartphone IMU sensors for reducing fear of fall (FoF) of a person
- Probability or proneness of one toward fall.

Index

A
Accelerometer, 10–16, 21, 25, 28, 29, 34, 39, 49–54, 57, 59, 69, 71–73, 75, 79, 80, 82, 87, 93, 94, 100–106, 108, 109, 113, 114, 120–130, 138–142
Alarm-fatigue, 141
Automatic feature extraction, 72, 80, 81, 99, 109

B
Blood pressure machine, 50, 54, 58, 59

C
Case study, 22, 125
Cloud, 3, 7–10, 14–16, 26, 27, 37, 42, 44–46, 65, 91, 114, 116, 133, 138
Cloud computing, 8, 15, 45, 46, 63, 69, 138, 139
Convolutional Neural Networks (CNN), 13, 43, 46, 70–76, 78–82, 89, 90, 99, 115, 116, 125, 126, 130, 140

D
Data fusion, 21, 33, 59, 62, 99, 102, 103, 105, 106, 109, 110, 126, 140, 141
Decision-level fusion, 62, 98, 99, 103, 105, 106
Deep Learning (DL), 1, 3, 7–9, 13, 18, 21, 26, 27, 42, 43, 45, 46, 61–63, 69–73, 75–83, 97, 99, 109, 115–117, 125, 126, 130, 138, 140, 141
Disease monitoring, 139
Disease prediction, 40, 50, 53, 65, 70, 97, 142

E
Edge computing, 14, 15, 44, 45, 63, 75, 141
Enabling technologies, 3, 25–27, 37, 46, 47, 69, 139

F
Fall detection, 2–5, 9, 10, 12, 18–22, 27, 42, 46, 62, 72, 75–77, 79, 87, 88, 90, 92–94, 104–106, 110, 117, 119, 126, 127, 131, 132, 137, 139–143
False-alarm, 31, 90, 93, 95, 141
Feature extraction, 2, 35, 36, 42, 69, 71, 73–75, 77–82, 88, 99, 100, 103, 109, 116, 120, 125, 130, 140
Feature fusion, 74, 99, 105, 106

G
Geriatric care, 5–7, 20, 29, 138
Gesture, 1, 29, 30, 32, 72, 123, 129, 130
Gyroscope, 11–16, 21, 25, 28, 29, 49–54, 57, 59, 69, 71, 72, 75, 79, 80, 82, 87, 94, 100–106, 108, 109, 113, 114, 120–128, 129, 138–142

H
Health monitoring, 3–5, 9, 10, 21, 27, 29, 30, 37, 50, 65, 70, 71, 73, 75, 97, 115, 119, 130, 138, 139, 141

S. Biswas, *Machine Learning and Deep Learning in Human Activity Recognition and Fall Detection*, Signals and Communication Technology,
https://doi.org/10.1007/978-3-032-09241-0

Health parameters, 5, 6, 9, 50, 54, 55, 57–59, 65, 139
Human Activity Recognition (HAR), 2–5, 10, 11, 13–22, 25–33, 35–38, 42–47, 50, 53, 57, 60–65, 69–83, 87, 88, 90–92, 95, 97, 98, 100–106, 109, 110, 113–117, 119–122, 124–131, 133, 134, 137–142

I
Imbalanced dataset, 60, 61, 106, 120
Information fusion, 98, 99, 110, 126, 140, 142
Internet of Things (IoT), 3, 7–10, 37, 42, 45, 46, 75, 90, 92, 93, 95, 97, 114, 129, 130, 133, 138, 139

L
Long Short-Term Memory (LSTM), 13, 44, 46, 70, 71, 73–76, 79, 81, 82, 89, 90, 99, 115, 125, 130, 140

M
Machine Learning (ML), 1, 3, 7–9, 12–14, 20, 21, 27, 33–36, 38, 40–43, 45, 46, 55–58, 61–64, 69, 70, 77, 82, 89, 95, 97, 99, 100, 105, 109, 113, 116, 117, 119, 125, 126, 129, 130, 138–142

O
Oximeter, 54, 58, 59, 139

P
Posture, 3, 4, 31, 33, 49, 70, 92–94, 101, 106, 127, 138
Prototype design, 94

R
Radar technology, 115, 138

S
Sensor, 3–16, 18–22, 25–37, 42–46, 49–54, 57–59, 61–65, 69–77, 79–82, 87, 88, 93–95, 97–110, 113–116, 119–131, 134, 138–143
Sensor fusion, 13, 21, 50, 59, 62, 70, 97, 98, 100, 101, 103, 104, 106, 108–110, 122, 123, 127, 139, 142
Sleeping, accelerometer, 109
Support Vector Machine (SVM), 13, 39, 42, 51, 53, 57, 88–90, 94, 97, 99, 100, 113, 126, 127, 129, 130, 140–142
Sustainable framework, 13, 14

MIX
Papier aus verantwortungsvollen Quellen
Paper from responsible sources
FSC® C105338

If you have any concerns about our products,
you can contact us on
ProductSafety@springernature.com

In case Publisher is established outside the EU,
the EU authorized representative is:
Springer Nature Customer Service Center GmbH
Europaplatz 3, 69115 Heidelberg, Germany

Printed by Libri Plureos GmbH
in Hamburg, Germany